LIVING
with
EXERCISE

Steven N. Blair, P.E.D.

Institute for Aerobics Research

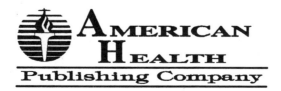

Library of Congress
    ISBN 1-878-513-04-4

Address orders to:

The LEARN® Education Center
1555 W. Mockingbird Lane, Suite 203
Dallas, Texas 75235

In Dallas (214) 637-7700
Or Toll Free (800) 736-7323
Fax Number (214) 637-0529

Permission to reprint cartoons was granted by the Universal Press Syndicate, Newspaper Enterprise Association, Tribune Media Services, King Features and the United Features Syndicate, Inc.

Cover design by Jay Colt Weesner

TABLE OF CONTENTS

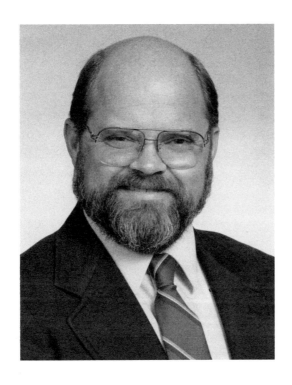

ABOUT THE AUTHOR

Steven N. Blair is Director of Epidemiology at the Institute for Aerobics Research in Dallas. Dr. Blair is a Fellow in the American College of Epidemiology, American College of Sports Medicine, Council on Cardiovascular Epidemiology, and American Academy of Physical Education. He is currently Vice President for Basic and Applied Sciences for the American College of Sports Medicine. His research focuses on the associations between lifestyle and health, with a specific emphasis on exercise, physical fitness, and chronic disease. He has published over 100 papers in the scientific literature. Dr. Blair was Chair of the Editorial Committee for the American College of Sports Medicine book, *Guidelines for Exercise Testing and Prescription*. He currently serves on the editorial boards of six scientific publications and on the Epidemiology and Disease Control study section at the National Institutes of Health. His research on physical fitness and mortality has been featured on the front pages of *The New York Times, USA Today*, and many other major newspapers; in *Newsweek, Time*, and *Sports Illustrated*; and on all three major TV networks.

INTRODUCTION

IS THIS BOOK FOR YOU

"I really should get more exercise."

"I remember that I seemed to feel better and had more energy a few years ago when I was more active and physically fit."

"I'm getting older and I really need to be more concerned about my health."

"I just seem to be tired all the time."

If you are having thoughts like these, then this book is for you. This book will teach you about the benefits of exercise, shape your beliefs and attitudes about exercise, and provide suggestions on how to integrate exercise into a busy 20th century lifestyle.

Surveys show that virtually all adult Americans believe that exercise is good for them. Yet the Centers for Disease Control, a branch of the U.S. Public Health Service, reports that less than 10% of adults exercise at the level recommended by the Surgeon General. Why is there such a tremendous gap between what people say they believe and their habits? I think one reason is the perception that most individuals have about what constitutes exercise. Think of it. When you see an advertisement on TV in which exercise is featured, what is the setting? Usually the characters are young, slim, beautiful, and athletic-looking. If you are like me, and most other people, you don't look like that. Most of us in the middle or later years are a little bit overweight, we have lost some or all of our hair, we have a few wrinkles, and we will not be mistaken for Tom Cruise or Michelle Pfeiffer. The point of all this is that we tend to think of exercise as being very vigorous and best done by young, athletic people.

Exercise is for all of us. Its benefits do not require athletic levels of fitness but can be achieved by virtually everyone with a modest exercise program. This is the good news. I hope that this book will change your view of what exercise is, of how you can improve your fitness and health, and feel better while doing it.

On the next page, please complete the "short quiz." It will help you determine if you are ready to make a positive change in your life and become a person who exercises. Be honest with yourself as you work through the quiz. Nobody else has to see your answers.

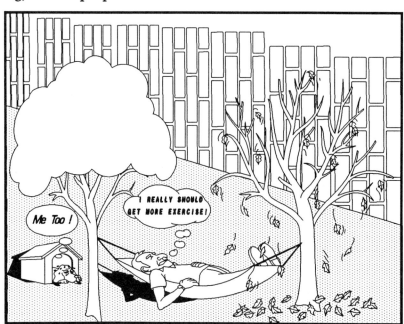

Short Quiz

1. Do you notice that you are
   not as fit as you used to be?   Yes   No

2. Do you believe that regular
   exercise is a good health habit?   Yes   No

3. Do you think you would feel
   better if you got more exercise?   Yes   No

4. Do you think that you must
   exercise vigorously to get
   benefits?   Yes   No

5. Does the idea of moderate
   exercise, such as walking,
   appeal to you?   Yes   No

If you answered any of these questions **YES,** then this book is for you. It will help you develop an exercise plan that is based on your personal beliefs, preferences, and daily schedule.

Can you no longer make ends meet, or are there other simple tasks that you now find hard to do?

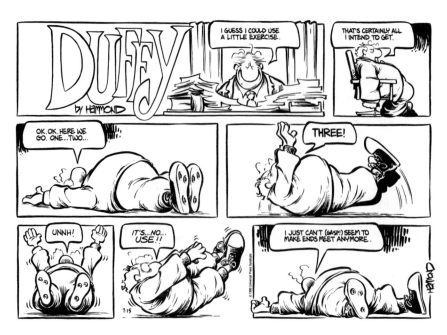

2

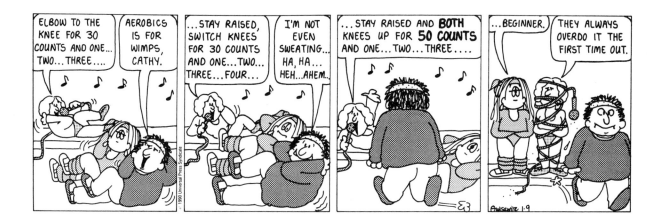

Do You Exercise Regularly?

If you currently exercise on a regular basis, you may think this book has nothing to offer you. Think again. Research has shown that a high percentage of exercisers drop out of their programs over time. Even people who have participated in supervised exercise classes and have become fit, frequently revert to their old sedentary habits. Why is this? I submit that it is because the exercise has not become fully integrated into their lifestyle, it is too much of an appendage, and it is easy to drop.

A major theme of this book is to help you build physical activity into your daily routine. If you can accomplish this goal, I believe you will be much more likely to maintain your activity program over time.

Many people believe that only vigorous, planned exercise, such as regular jogging or an aerobics class, provide health and functional benefits. This book will help dispel that myth. Building routine and moderate physical activity into your life can make a difference.

HOW THIS BOOK IS DIFFERENT

This book is unlike other exercise books or exercise programs you have read. Most other exercise books fall into two categories. The most predominant type of exercise book gives detailed information about a specific exercise prescription you should follow. You are told about target heart rates, frequency of exercise, length of exercise session, and precisely what type of exercise you should do. Frequently, lists of specific exercises are given with a detailed plan for several weeks. Another feature of this type of book or program is its emphasis on relatively high-intensity activity. "No pain, no gain" or "Go for the burn" are the type of statements frequently seen. These books often appear designed to get people fit for Olympic competition or at least develop their maximum athletic ability.

The second type of exercise book promises more than it can deliver, and many such books are outright frauds. These books capitalize on some people's dislike of exercise and promise fitness and health without exercise. "Fitness in a 30-second workout" or "Become fit in 15 minutes a week" are typical examples of statements from fraudulent books.

Exercise scientists have learned a lot about the scientific basis for exercise prescription over the past 30 years, and this information can be used to specify an exercise program as some books do. This approach, however, is too regimented. It ignores the reality of how many individuals view exercise and the complications of fitting a regimented program into their daily schedules. Furthermore, recent studies have

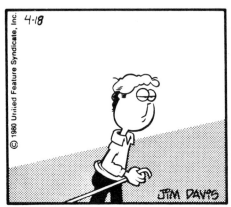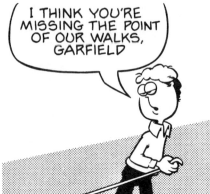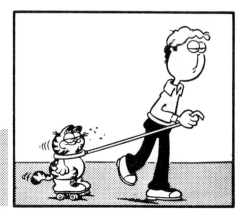

shown that the intensity and dose of exercise, defined in the typical exercise prescription, are more than is needed to get important health benefits.

The fraudulent books also miss the point. It **does** take a certain amount of exercise to improve physical fitness and to enhance health. And, as for other life goals, you can't expect health and fitness benefits without some effort. I think that these "no-effort exercise" books have a useful feature, and that is the concept that exercise can be integrated into your daily habits without a major disruption of your schedule.

I describe an approach to exercise in this book that falls between the extremes of a highly structured, detailed program and a false promise of fitness without effort. I will show you that moderate levels of exercise have an enormous health benefit. You can increase the amount of energy you expend, calories you burn, and improve your fitness with minimal disruption of your day.

Take the Dare

I will make exercise so unintimidating and easy to build into your life that you will have no reason not to increase your activity. **I dare you** not to think differently about exercise after you read this book. **I dare you** to have fun, feel better, do more, look better, and live longer by incorporating a modest amount of exercise into your daily schedule.

A Different Approach

There are several major differences between this and other exercise books. This book:

- **Emphasizes moderate-intensity, lifestyle activities.** Most exercise books tell you about target heart rate, working above the aerobic threshold and going for the burn, and they generally stress vigorous physical activity. There is nothing wrong with that approach; indeed, it is essential if you are training for competitive athletics. But most of us do not need such vigorous exercise for adequate fitness or to produce significant health benefits. In fact, sedentary individuals need do no more difficult exercise than taking a brisk walk in order to get important health and fitness benefits.

- **Takes a behavioral, problem-solving approach.** Other books on exercise give you detailed recommendations on the type of activity and the frequency, intensity and duration of your workout. This advice is fine for some, but I find that most people do better if they participate in formulating their individual exercise plans. You are the one who has to make the plan work; you are the one who must make changes in your schedule and exercise behavior. I will give you some of the principles you should apply and offer some practical suggestions on getting started and overcoming problems, but you must get involved in making and following an exercise plan.

This book also includes many suggestions for getting around mental and physical roadblocks that might get in your way as you are starting out.

- **Focuses on lifestyle activities.** The recommendations presented here concentrate more on lifestyle activities than on sports or typical exercise regimens. Most people are busy with work, family, and home responsibilities. You are more likely to increase your exercise if you can make it more a part of your daily routine and take it in short bouts than if you have to find an hour and go to a gym.

EXERCISE BOOM OR BUST

Why a book about exercise? Isn't everyone active these days? Those of you who are middle-aged or older can remember when you never saw a jogger on the street and racquetball clubs and aerobics dance classes were nonexistent. National surveys by the U.S Public Health Service confirm that more adults are exercising today than they were 20 or more years ago, but there is still a long way to go.

As much as 30% of our adult population is almost totally sedentary, and the exercise boom has not been equally distributed. Young men are quite active as a group, while older women are the most inactive. White collar and professional individuals are more likely to engage in regular exercise than blue collar workers.

This book has been developed to help those who are inactive to become at least moderately active. I will not focus much on high level activity and formal vigorous exercise programs. People who are interested in such programs or who become interested as a result of becoming more active should consult an exercise professional or a book that gives detailed advice on exercise prescription.

In this book, you will learn how to evaluate carefully your level of physical activity and physical fitness. This will require some record-keeping and a few simple calculations, but it is not difficult. You will be asked to chart your behavior and record your progress. If recording and charting are not for you, this book is still valuable and will give you some information and ideas for becoming more active. The emphasis is on building moderate physical activity into your life, so you expend more energy and become more physically fit.

WHAT YOU CAN LEARN FROM THIS BOOK

I realize that information alone is not sufficient to produce changes in behavior, but I do believe that it has an important role. This is probably a bias coming from my 20 years as a university professor. I think that you are more likely to make good decisions about your physical activity habits if you are well informed. In this first part of the book, I offer some basic information about health and the human body.

The Human Energy Machine. The human body is a wonderful engine, superbly designed to transform the energy in food to a form that the body can use to move, think, grow, and maintain life's functions. As long as we are alive, our bodies are constantly converting energy. All of this energy comes from the food we eat. It is ultimately combined with oxygen to liberate the energy used by the body's cells to carry out their functions. A major focus of this book is on the body's energy balance: energy from food and energy spent in the body's various metabolic processes.

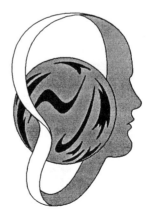

Physical activity is nothing more than a way to increase energy expenditure. Exercise does not have to be vigorous to spend energy. Standing uses more than sitting, and moving about burns more calories than standing. Brisk walking takes more energy than casual activity around the home or office, and running or strenuous sports uses still more energy.

This book will also provide you with many suggestions for increasing energy expenditure. While this can be achieved by a formal exercise prescription or participation in an aerobics class, the emphasis here will be on ways you can build opportunities into your daily life to burn more calories, become healthier, and more physically fit.

Use It or Lose It. A great advantage the body has over other machines is that it is not worn out by use. In general, body parts and systems function better when they are kept active. Muscles shrink and become weak with disuse; so does the heart. Your joints function better if you are physically active. They have thicker cartilage between the bones, and they have more lubricating fluid. Even the mind seems to suffer from disuse.

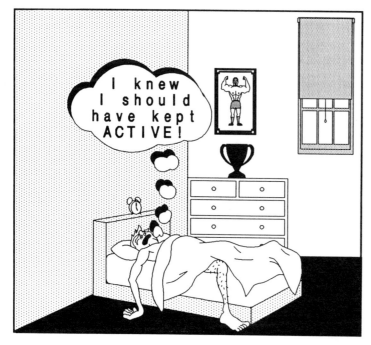

Studies in which volunteers have stayed in bed for several weeks highlight the effects of inactivity. The bones lose mineral and become weak, the heart cannot pump as much blood, muscles weaken, and overall physical fitness declines. Prolonged space flight has the same effect. Astronauts rapidly become deconditioned. There is little room to exercise and move around in a space capsule or the shuttle, and there is no force of gravity to work against. One of the major challenges of prolonged space flight is to keep the astronauts fit enough to walk away from the shuttle after it lands. The decline in fitness and other aspects of physiological function is so severe that space travel has been referred to as accelerated aging. Fortunately, some of the ill effects can be lessened by an exercise program in space. The fitness losses are rapidly reversed after the astronauts return to earth and resume normal activities.

It is possible to exercise too much and put undue stress on some parts of the body. This can cause problems. But for the vast majority of us, we rust out rather than wear out.

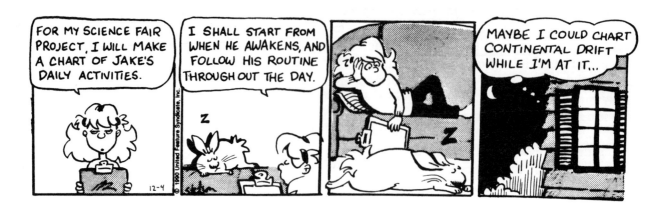

6

Exercise Benefits

Hundreds of research studies over the past few decades have demonstrated clearly the health benefits of regular physical activity. The evidence has become compelling. There are skeptics who claim that exercise has no health value, of course. But then, there is also a flat earth society and the Tobacco Institute says that there is no evidence that smoking is bad for you! In subsequent chapters, I will review some of the evidence on the benefits and risks of exercise.

Building a More Active Lifestyle

Being physically active must be somewhat difficult or there wouldn't be so many sedentary people. It is certainly not impossible, because there are millions who have changed their exercise habits. The physically active lifestyle presented here is less formidable to adopt than some other exercise programs you may have used before. So give it a try.

The following chapters will help you move through the "stages of change" that will help you to become more active. These changes are listed below:

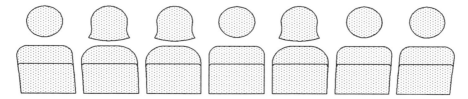

STAGES OF CHANGE
1. Start thinking about changing
2. Clarify attitudes and beliefs
3. Get started
4. Stick with it
5. Maintain an acceptable level of activity
6. Anticipate and overcome problems and barriers

HOW TO USE THIS BOOK

The main purpose of this book is to help you design your personal program of physical activity and to help you implement the plan so that you can become more healthy and fit. If you hire an architect to design your new house, he or she will ask you questions and try to learn as much about you as possible. This will help the expert create a design for your house that fits your lifestyle and gives you pleasure. In the case of physical activity, I am asking you to become your own expert, and design a program that will work for you.

Have you ever successfully changed a health behavior in the past? Perhaps you started flossing your teeth regularly or began wearing your seat belt while in a car. What prompted you to change? Did a health professional recommend it? Did a friend or family member convince you? Did you read an article and decide to change? Or, did you think about the negative health consequences of your behavior and decide to make changes?

Analyze these past successes. What caused you to decide to change? How did you go about making the change? What factors contributed to your success? What problems did you overcome in making the change? Think about it - perhaps you are more of an expert in health behavior change than you thought. Can you use some of the strategies for making changes that have been helpful in the past to help you increase your physical activity level?

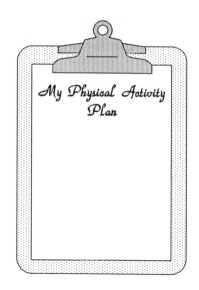

There are several other questions you should ask yourself about how to design your physical activity program. What activities do you like? What activities have you had success with in the past? How much time are you willing to invest in improving your physical fitness and health? What is your current lifestyle? A thoughtful review of these issues and specific answers to these questions will help you begin to plan your new lifestyle. In developing your plan, you should carefully consider the following:

1. **Set realistic goals for physical activity.**

2. **Develop a sensible plan for implementation.**

3. **Learn to avoid pitfalls.**

4. **Use this book to help you lead a healthy and active life.**

You do not have to read this book from start to finish in order to plan your physical activity. Individuals have different knowledge and beliefs about exercise, differ in their motivation to make changes, and vary on the types of obstacles they need to overcome. Furthermore, different approaches to health behavior change will be used by different people. There is nothing wrong with reading the book straight through, but I offer a few suggestions on how you can pick and choose parts that may be of use to you as you attempt to change.

- If you are currently unfit, unhealthy, or are middle-aged or older, you may benefit from Chapter 1, especially the sections on "When to stop exercise," "Do I need a medical exam?" and the "Physical Activity Readiness Questionnaire." The Chapter 2 sections on fitness appraisal may also be helpful.

- If you respond best when you know the scientific evidence for a health behavior, check the information in Chapter 1.

- If you hate to exercise, it might help to review the section on advantages and disadvantages of exercise in Chapter 1.

- Consider your history of health behavior change. If information is what makes you change, read Chapter 1. If you like a logical, sequential, and behavioral approach, reading through Chapters 1, 2, 3, and 4 may be best for you. You need not, and probably should not, read them straight through in one sitting. Read, reflect, try out some of the suggestions, then perhaps revise and try again. Then, go on to the next chapter.

- If you think your ability to change is related to social and environmental factors, read Chapters 3 and 7.

- If lack of time is a major barrier to increasing your physical activity, check the sections in Chapter 3 on "Seek opportunities to spend energy" and "The 2-minute walk."

MY PLAN FOR USING THIS BOOK

Take the time now to scan the chapter outline. Think about the issues mentioned above, analyze your own situation, and skim through some of the chapters to get a general idea of the contents. Then, develop your plan on how to use this book to your advantage. What chapters will you read first? What chapters might be the most helpful for you? Write down the main features of your plan on the form provided on the next page. Use this as your guide. The following sample plan may be helpful.

MY PLAN FOR USING THIS BOOK

(Sample)

Chapters To Read	Date For Completion	Comments
1	03-07	Complete PAR-Q , Take quiz
1	03-08	List advantages / disadvantages
2	03-12	Complete charts, Take tests
3	03-17	Complete plan for change - complete lists
4	03-29	Evaluate activity level - complete lists
5	04-01	Monitor food intake - 4 food groups ?
6	04-07	Increase exercise level
7	04-07	Start 5-minute walks - walking club?
8	04-14	Family activity check
9	04-28	10-minute walks - Review!

MY PLAN FOR USING THIS BOOK

Chapters To Read	Date For Completion	Comments

Chapter 1

THINKING ABOUT IT

IS ACTIVITY GOOD FOR ME

"Should I increase my physical activity?"

"Will it really be good for me?"

"What is the health value of becoming more physically active?"

Surveys show that most Americans believe that regular physical activity is a good health habit. There are a lot of misconceptions about exercise and physical activity. In this section we will review some of the research evidence on physical activity and health. If you are already knowledgeable about physical activity and health, you may wish to scan the next few pages.

THE ANTHROPOLOGY OF PHYSICAL ACTIVITY

Humans are marvelous endurance animals and physical activity is a natural aspect of the human condition. It is not something artificial or unusual that 20th century men and women developed to occupy their leisure time. Physical activity has played a significant role in human development.

Early Humans

Humans have been on this planet for at least 2 million years. For 99.5% of that time, we existed as nomads and survived by hunting and gathering food. Studies of the few remaining groups of

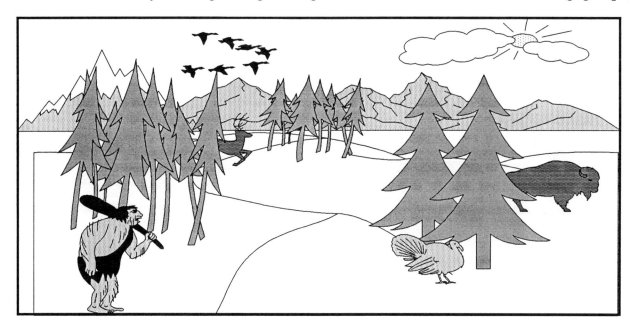

hunter/gatherers have provided us with some insight into the way of life followed by our ancestors. The nomadic way of life required large outlays of energy. Small bands or families roamed the grassy plains of the temperate zone, following animals and gathering seeds, roots, and fruit. The only mode of transportation was walking, and all possessions had to be carried.

Our ancestors spent energy at a moderate rate. Hunters walked, trailing their prey, and if they were successful, carried the meat back to the camp with them. The hunts frequently extended over several days and many miles. After a successful hunt, it might be several days before it was necessary to go out again. During these intervals, time spent in camp probably involved low levels of physical activity. Inevitably, stocks had to be replenished, and the hunters had to return to the field. This cycle occurred with regularity, so the people stayed physically fit.

The gathering of food also required hours of moderate energy expenditure. Many times, gatherers would have to travel several miles from the camp to collect food. Then, of course, they had to carry it back.

Life of the nomads was relatively slow-paced. Although they spent much of their time relaxing in camp and in light recreational activities, they also were moderately active for several hours a week. That was enough to keep them physically fit. In fact, modern studies of remaining hunter/gatherers show physical fitness levels 25 to 50% higher than those of residents of industrialized countries. This supports the notion that the nomadic lifestyle promotes the development and maintenance of physical fitness.

Disease was rare among early humans. Modern chronic problems, such as heart disease, were unknown. The small bands in which people lived were not large enough to sustain a pool of infectious diseases. Most deaths were probably due to starvation when food was scarce, accidents, natural disasters, violence, and old age.

For almost the entire period of human history, our ancestors have had vastly different lifestyles than we do now. We evolved as creatures well adapted to a nomadic existence; but not very well suited to the stressful, crowded, sedentary, pollution-filled, abundant-calorie lifestyle of the modern world. We do not tolerate this way of life very well. Our high rates of heart disease, cancer, diabetes, and other health problems attest to this.

The Agricultural Period

About 10,000 years ago, human beings began to domesticate plants and animals. They stopped wandering across large geographical areas and settled in fertile valleys suited to growing crops. Animals were domesticated and grazed on pastures near the settlements. More permanent homes were built, and villages and towns developed. Workers began to specialize with some assuming the responsibility for producing food for all.

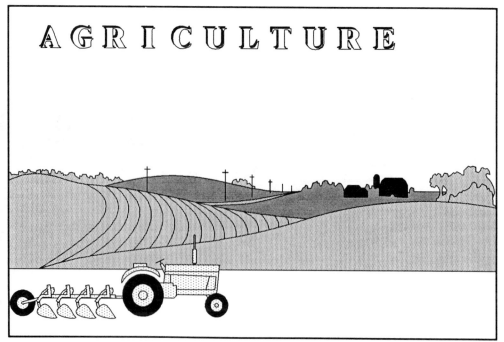

Daily energy expenditure during the agricultural period was high, even for those not working on farms. Most of the transportation was still by foot, and many occupational and household tasks were accomplished by human power. Physical demands on agricultural workers may have been even greater than on the nomads. Farming probably required more hours a day than hunting and gathering. Digging in the soil is harder work than trailing game or gathering fruit.

The major health problem during this period was starvation. As people congregated in larger and larger groups, infectious disease became more prevalent. Toward the latter part of the agricultural period, after cities had developed, infectious disease became a major health problem. The most striking example, of course, is the plagues in Europe during the Middle Ages. Modern chronic disease was still rare, but probably occurred in wealthier individuals who had access to richer diets and led more sedentary lifestyles. Wars and other forms of violence took an increasing toll on human lives.

Lifestyle during the agricultural period was undergoing rapid and major changes - and humans who had evolved from a nomadic existence were forced into vastly different environments.

The Industrial Period

The industrial period covers from the middle of the 18th century to the middle of the 20th century. This period is marked by the development of steam, and later, internal combustion engines to provide power for transportation and manufacturing. During this time, people congregated more and more in cities, although there was still a large rural population. Farm workers and city dwellers alike had physically active lifestyles. While some segments of society were relatively inactive, the middle-class and professionals spent more energy in the routine activities of daily living than is true today. Most bankers and lawyers in large cities lived a few blocks from their offices and walked to work. Furnaces had to be stoked, the horses cared for, and most household tasks required human power.

INDUSTRIALIZATION

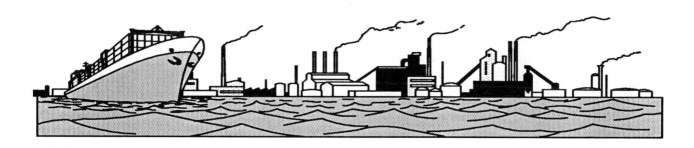

Even well into the 20th century, most individuals in the industrialized world spent more calories each day than we do today. The average daily caloric intake in the U.S. was higher in 1900 than it is now, but Americans today are heavier. If caloric intake has decreased, and Americans have become heavier, the logical explanation is that levels of energy expenditure have fallen.

During the industrial period, health problems also changed. Starvation was not eliminated, but became much less of a problem. Infectious diseases were the leading cause of death, even as late as the first part of this century. Our lifestyle resembled less and less that of our nomadic forebears.

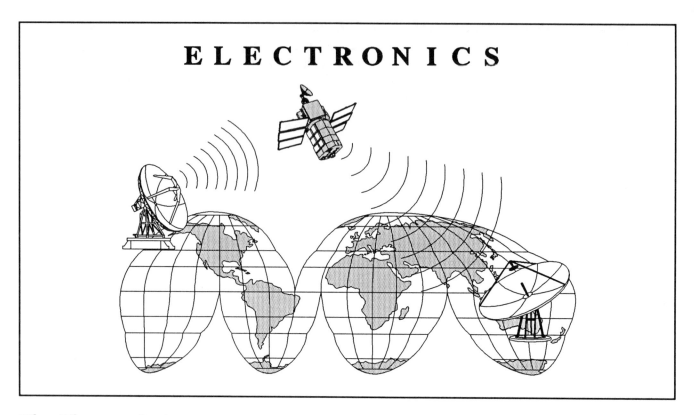

ELECTRONICS

The Electronic Age

Enormous technological and social changes have occurred in the latter half of the 20th century. Urbanization, the increased use of electrical power to provide comforts, greater wealth for many, and the computer revolution have drastically altered our lives. The widespread availability of inexpensive fast food, high in calories and fat, more and more sedentary leisure-time activities, such as television, and labor-saving devices at work and at home have had profound effects on energy intake and expenditure.

Today, chronic diseases are the major causes of death in the industrialized world. Approximately 70% of all deaths in the U.S. are due to cardiovascular disease and cancer. The causes of these diseases are primarily related to lifestyle. Leading problems include diets high in fat, salt, and calories; cigarette smoking; and physical inactivity. You and I cannot adapt quickly to these conditions. Humans are obviously not going to return to a nomadic way of life, however, positive changes can be made that will help make our lifestyles more active and natural. In later chapters, I will provide some recommendations to help you engineer more physical activity back into your life.

RESEARCH ON PHYSICAL ACTIVITY AND HEALTH

Scholars and philosophers since ancient times have commented on the health value of regular exercise.

"All parts of the body which have a function, if used in moderation and exercised in labours in which each is accustomed, become thereby healthy, well-developed and age more slowly, but if unused and left idle, they become liable to disease, defective in growth, and age quickly."

Hippocrates

The "Exercise Hypothesis"

Modern research has shown that Hippocrates was right. More than 30 years ago, Dr. Jeremy Morris observed that heart disease death rates were lower in London bus conductors than in the bus drivers. He attributed this to the increased physical activity of the conductors, who climbed up the stairs to collect fares in the double-decker buses. The drivers were more sedentary and spent most of their day sitting. This study is considered the modern research that led to the "exercise hypothesis," which states that physical activity may protect against the development of heart disease.

Many other studies over the past three decades have clarified and strengthened the exercise hypothesis. Lower death rates have been seen in workers with more active jobs. For instance, longshoremen who unload ships were less likely to die than the clerks and foremen who worked alongside them. Railroad section hands lived longer than their bosses and other railroad workers in sedentary jobs. Higher levels of physical activity during leisure time have been associated with lower death rates in college alumni and in British executive grade civil servants.

The findings from these studies are not due to the influences of other well-known health risk factors, such as cigarette smoking, high blood pressure, high blood cholesterol, and obesity. A summary of these studies suggests that physical inactivity is as important as these other risk factors. And since sedentary living habits are so common, they constitute a major public health problem.

The Aerobics Center Longitudinal Study

Our research group has followed patients who received preventive medical examinations at The Aerobics Center in Dallas. More than 10,000 men and 3,000 women were examined between 1970 and 1982. During follow up to 1985, 240 men and 43 women died. All patients in the study were given an exercise test on a treadmill during their examinations to determine the maximum physical effort they could give. We examined the relationship of this measure of physical fitness to the risk of dying during the follow-up period. Patients with low levels of physical fitness were much more likely to die than those in the moderate or high-fitness categories. Death rates for cardiovascular disease, cancer, and for all causes combined are shown in the graphs on the following page. Rates for the low-fitness group are in black, the moderate-fitness group rates are shown by the bars with diagonal lines, and the high-fitness group rates are indicated by the bars with the grid design.

There was a tremendous drop in death rates from the low to the moderate fitness categories, with some further improvement for those in the high fitness group. For example, women in the low fitness group had an all-cause death rate of 40 per 10,000, moderately fit women had a death rate of 16 per 10,000, and the rate for the high fit women was only 7 per 10,000.

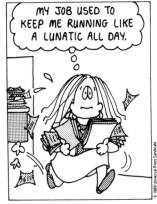
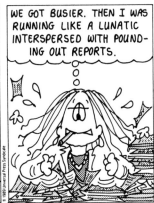
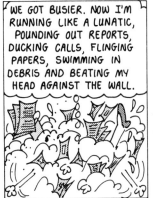
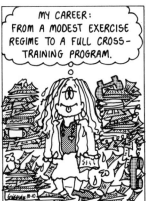

Death Rates By Fitness Groups, Women

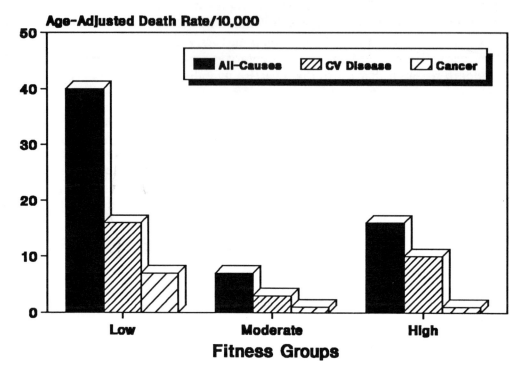

Death Rates By Fitness Groups, Men

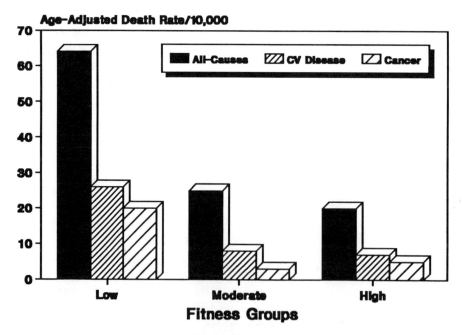

The great benefit in being out of the low fit group is the most important finding of the study. You do not have to be an Olympic champion to receive health benefits from physical fitness. The moderate level of fitness can be achieved by almost all middle-aged and older men and women with a modest exercise program. In fact, the primary message of this book is based on the observation that a moderate level of fitness seems to provide significant health benefits. You do not have to become a marathon runner, or even run at all, to make a major impact on your health. I will show you later how to increase your daily energy expenditure to achieve a protective level of fitness.

Acute Versus Chronic Activity

There is more good news. Recent research indicates that exercise provides some immediate benefits. You do not have to wait several weeks for a training effect to occur. For example, a single exercise session makes your muscle cells more sensitive to insulin. This has important implications for diabetics or for those who are prone to diabetes and have high levels of blood sugar. When muscle cells absorb insulin more readily, they are better able to draw sugar out of the blood and use it for fuel for contraction. A single bout of exercise also improves your ability to break down blood clots. This may help prevent a clot from blocking a vital artery in the heart or brain and lessen your risk of a heart attack or stroke.

A single brief session of moving about frequently makes you feel better as well. If you have been sitting for some time working at your desk, a short walk of even a few minutes invigorates you. I have frequently had people, participating in exercise training studies, tell me they felt better when they returned for the second session. Some of this effect may be psychological rather than physiological, but it is real nevertheless.

HOW MUCH PHYSICAL ACTIVITY DO I NEED

You may be familiar with the traditional "exercise prescription" as described by the American College of Sports Medicine and other scientific or professional groups. The prescription can be summarized as follows:

Exercise frequency -- You should exercise three to five times a week.

Exercise intensity -- You should exercise at 65 to 90% of your maximum heart rate.

Exercise duration -- You should exercise for 20 to 40 minutes each session.

This approach is based on dozens of exercise training studies that have been conducted over the past two or three decades. This advice is scientifically sound in most respects, but it does have some problems. First, it is based on relatively short-term studies; few were longer than six months. The objective of these studies was to see how much exercise is required to improve maximum oxygen uptake. The results of these studies do not necessarily apply when a long-term perspective and health outcomes are considered. If we are interested in how much exercise we need over a lifetime in order to be healthy, the exercise prescription approach may not provide the best answer.

A second problem with the exercise prescription method is that it encourages you to think of physical activity as a dichotomy. That is, you are either sedentary or active, and there is no middle ground. This may discourage many people who find that they cannot adhere to the strict guidelines of the prescription. They may consider themselves failures and stop exercising altogether.

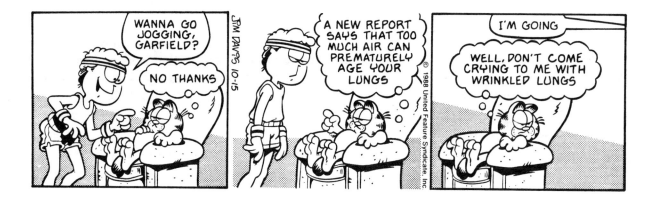

17

I would like for you to think of physical activity as a continuum, from people who spend all day in bed to high-level endurance athletes. The members of the first group spend most of their day at rest, and they have a very low daily energy expenditure. Athletes or people in very physically demanding jobs have a much higher energy expenditure than people who are sedentary.

The data from our study of physical fitness and death, reviewed earlier, clearly shows a gradual decline in death rates across fitness categories. Being moderately fit is much better than being low fit. Our results are consistent with studies on physical activity and health. **My conclusion is that doing <u>something</u> is better than doing <u>nothing</u>.** Standing is better than sitting, moving around is better than standing, and walking is better than just moving around.

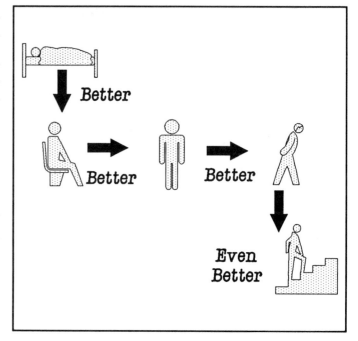

A good exercise prescription for the 30 to 50 million mostly sedentary and unfit Americans is "turn off the television, get up off your fanny, go out the door, and move around a bit." We have learned from research that it doesn't matter what you do. Any activity that increases your metabolic rate and burns more calories can provide benefits.

IS EXERCISE SAFE FOR ME

Exercise is a good health habit, but there are some precautions that need to be remembered. Persons considering an increase in their physical activity should carefully review the benefits and ways to minimize the risks.

Does Exercise "Wear Out" My Heart?

One of the most persistent myths about exercise is that it somehow "wears out" your heart. Some have even gone so far as to say that a person only has a fixed number of heartbeats allocated at birth, and when they are used, you die. Advocates of this myth believe that since your heart rate increases with exercise, you are shortening your length of life.

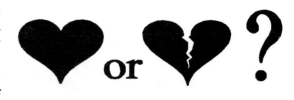

There is absolutely no scientific evidence to support this view. But, even if it were true, exercise would delay death. Active and fit individuals have lower heart rates at rest and during all types of routine daily activities. The difference can be 10 to 20 beats a minute or more, and at that rate, you would "save" thousands of beats each day. Your heart rate does increase during vigorous exercise, but the total "extra" beats during exercise are far fewer than the "saved" beats due to increased physical fitness.

Exercise actually strengthens the heart. The muscle fibers become thicker and stronger; the fit heart has a greater muscle mass than an unfit, flabby one. The more powerful heart can pump more blood with each beat. Also, the fit heart has more reserve capacity. It is more likely to continue to provide adequate circulation to sustain life, even if you suffer a heart attack.

Sudden Death During Exercise

About 350,000 people in the U.S. die of a heart attack each year before they reach a hospital. In about one-half of these cases, the victims had no warning and no prior history of heart disease. This characteristic of sudden and unexpected death, in an apparently healthy person, is perhaps the most frightening feature of heart disease.

Some sudden and unexpected deaths do occur during exercise. One such example is the highly publicized, sudden death of Jim Fixx, author of *The Complete Book of Running*. Occasionally, sudden death occurs in a young, highly-fit athlete, but fortunately this tragedy is quite rare. Does exercise cause sudden death? Several points must be considered in seeking an answer to this question.

- Sudden death occurs during all types of activity: driving a car, eating lunch, taking a shower, and any other example you can think of. Only a fraction of sudden deaths occur during exercise.

- In virtually all cases of sudden death, including the death of Jim Fixx, the victims had significant heart disease or abnormalities. The disease killed them, not the exercise. Even if exercise precipitated the event, the tragedy was imminent anyway.

- If exercise causes sudden death, we would not expect to find lower death rates in more physically active and fit groups as reviewed earlier in this chapter.

- If exercise does cause sudden death but also provides protection against other causes of death, we need to consider the overall cost/benefit ratio. One important study in Seattle a few years ago found that regular exercisers had a slightly increased risk of sudden death during the times they were engaged in vigorous activity. Overall, however, **sedentary** men were about three times more likely to experience sudden death than the men who were regular exercisers. Thus, it seems clear that regular exercise prevents more sudden death than it causes.

In summary, there is an increased risk of sudden death during vigorous physical activity, but the health benefits appear to far outweigh the risks. The best way to reduce your risk of sudden death is to follow good health practices to prevent heart disease, since that is what causes most cases of sudden death. Avoid the use of tobacco, follow a low-fat and low-cholesterol diet, maintain a normal blood pressure, and maintain at least a moderate level of physical activity.

Exercise-Related Injuries

Some people may avoid physical activity because they are afraid of injuring themselves. Statements such as, "Every runner I know is always injured," and "Aerobic dance is sure hard on your feet and legs," are common. There has been a good deal of publicity about exercise-related injuries in the popular media and in professional publications. In my opinion, there has been considerable over-reaction and myths abound. We should again consider the cost/benefit ratio for physical activity. If you spend the rest of your life in bed, you will probably never have an exercise-related injury. But, the costs and harmful effects of inactivity are not worth the loss of benefits from not exercising.

The risk of exercise-related injuries is not high. Our research shows that if 100 sedentary individuals were to enroll in an aerobics class and

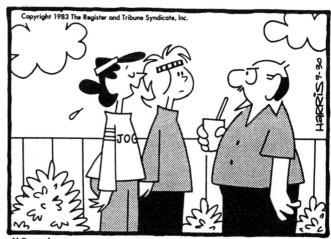

"Stanley exercises religiously. Does one push-up and thanks God it didn't kill him."

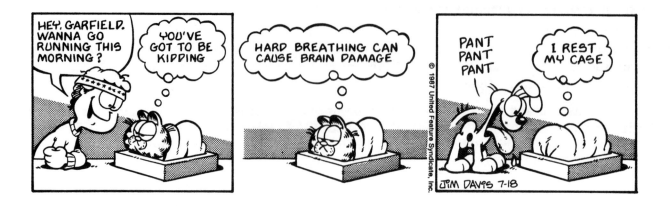

participate for one year, 10 to 15 would have some type of bone, muscle, or joint injury due to the exercise. And in this example, injury is defined as having a problem that would cause you to stop exercising for at least seven days. Most injuries are not very serious and you can recover with only a few days rest.

In our studies at the Institute, we also found that in a large group of runners who were averaging about 10 to 12 miles of running per week, no more than 2 to 3 % a year reported injuries serious enough to seek medical care. Our research also shows that a significant number of injuries occur in sedentary persons as well as exercisers, so being inactive does not guarantee freedom from injuries.

Very little is known about how to prevent exercise-related injuries. Many exercise leaders give a lot of advice about injury prevention, but it is not firmly based on research studies. The two major predictors of injury are how much you exercise and whether you have had a previous injury. There is also reason to believe that more vigorous activity carries a higher risk of injury. We see little difference in injury risk between men and women or between older and younger individuals, so there seems to be no reason to avoid physical activity because of your age or sex.

The risk of exercise-related injury appears to be low, at least within the range of activity recommended in this book. Injury rates are also lower in walkers when compared to runners or those who participate in vigorous sports. If you become more enthusiastic and start running dozens of miles a week, injury risk will increase. If you follow the advice given in this book, serious injury should not be a major problem.

When to Stop Exercise

Exercise is a normal human activity and is quite safe for most people. Problems can arise during exercise, however, and you need to know what signs and symptoms you need to be concerned about.

For instance, it is normal to breathe more frequently and more deeply while exercising. Your heart will beat faster, and you may begin to flush and perspire. These signs are normal and should not cause you to become alarmed. There are some signs and symptoms, however, that could indicate the need to slow down, stop, or even seek a medical opinion.

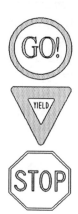

A heart attack is potentially the most serious problem that can arise during exercise. The most common indication of a heart attack in an uncomfortable feeling of pressure, pain, fullness, or squeezing in the center of the chest behind the breastbone. This sensation may radiate to the neck, jaw, shoulder, or arm. If you notice this feeling during exercise, you should stop and sit or lie down. If the pain goes away in one or two minutes, you might try to duplicate it by moving your arms and trunk. If you can reproduce the feeling in this manner, it is probably not of heart origin - it could be pain in your joints or muscles - and you may resume exercise.

If the chest discomfort does not go away in one or two minutes, you should seek emergency assistance. The common reaction to a heart attack is denial, and you should not tell yourself that it is only gas or some other minor problem. When in doubt, call your doctor, contact an emergency service, or go to an emergency room. If the discomfort goes away shortly after you stop exercise, but resumes with repeated exercise, you should contact your doctor. Increased respiration during exercise is normal, but extreme shortness of breath with mild to moderate activity is not.

If you take your pulse immediately after exercise and notice a lot of "skipped" beats, or if you feel a lot of "skipped" beats in your chest that are confirmed by taking your pulse, you should call your doctor. Some "skipped" heart beats are normal and occur in most of us. Do not be alarmed if you occasionally experience them.

Severe nausea, fatigue, slow recovery, or lightheadedness with mild or moderate exercise is abnormal and you should contact a doctor about these symptoms.

Most of the signs and symptoms listed above can be either a potential problem or the body's normal response to exercise. It is often difficult for most individuals and sometimes even difficult for a doctor to recognize a problem. You should not be a hypochondriac but you should not be too stoic either. Listen carefully to your body. Does the response seem normal? Is it something you recall noticing in the past? Is it a new sensation? Be alert for denial, and when in doubt, seek a medical review.

DO I NEED A MEDICAL EXAM

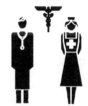

Do I Need a Medical Exam?

This is one of the questions most frequently asked in connection with starting an exercise program. The most conservative response is that anyone over 40 to 45 years of age should check with their doctor before starting an exercise program. But this simplistic advice is not ideal. There are tens of millions of sedentary adults in the U.S. If they all went to their doctors for recommendations about exercise, the medical practice system would break down. Requiring a medical examination before starting to exercise also presents a significant barrier to changing your physical activity habits. Lack of money or time may deter some people from seeing their doctor and give them a ready excuse to delay a physical activity program.

I believe that most sedentary adults in this country can safely get up off their couches and move around a bit without obtaining medical clearance. However, you should be prudent. If you are not healthy, and you are middle-aged or older and plan to engage in vigorous exercise, then a medical examination is recommended. In the following sections, you will learn how to decide whether or not you need a medical evaluation prior to increasing your physical activity.

PHYSICAL ACTIVITY READINESS QUESTIONNAIRE

The Physical Activity Readiness Questionnaire or PAR-Q was developed in Canada by the British Columbia Ministry of Health as part of an effort to increase the public's activity levels. It is a simple, self-administered checklist that can help you decide if you need to consult with your doctor prior to changing your physical activity habits. The PAR-Q is presented on the next page. Take a few moments to complete the questions and follow the recommendations. This will help you to determine if you should see a physician before continuing with your exercise program.

The Physical Activity Readiness Questionnaire

PAR-Q is designed to help you help yourself. Many health benefits are associated with regular exercise, and the completion of PAR-Q is a sensible first step to take if you are planning to increase the amount of physical activity in your life.

For most people physical activity should not pose any problem or hazard. PAR-Q has been designed to identify the small number of adults for whom physical activity might be inappropriate or those who should have medical advice concerning the type of activity most suitable for them.

Common sense is your best guide in answering these few questions. Please read them carefully and circle the YES or NO for each question as it applies to you.

1.	Has your doctor ever said you have heart trouble?	YES	NO
2.	Do you frequently have pains in your heart and chest?	YES	NO
3.	Do you often feel faint or have spells of severe dizziness?	YES	NO
4.	Has a doctor ever said your blood pressure was too high?	YES	NO
5.	Has your doctor ever told you that you have a bone or joint problem, such as arthritis, that has been aggravated by exercise, or might be made worse with exercise?	YES	NO
6.	Is there a good physical reason, not mentioned here, why you should not follow an activity program even if you wanted to?	YES	NO
7.	Are you over age 65 and not accustomed to vigorous exercise?	YES	NO

If you answered YES to one or more questions:

If you have not recently done so, consult with your personal physician by telephone or in person **BEFORE** increasing your physical activity and/or taking a fitness test. Tell him or her what questions you answered YES.

After a medical evaluation, seek advice from your physician as to your suitability for:
- unrestricted physical activity, probably on a gradually increasing basis or
- restricted and supervised activity to meet your specific needs, at least on an initial basis. Check in your community for special programs or services.

If you answered NO to all questions:

If you answered the questions on the PAR-Q accurately, you have reasonable assurance of your present suitability for:
- A GRADUATED EXERCISE PROGRAM--A gradual increase in proper exercise promotes good fitness development while minimizing or eliminating discomfort.
- AN EXERCISE TEST--Simple tests of fitness may be undertaken if you so desire.

Postpone exercise or exercise testing:

- If you have a temporary minor illness, such as a common cold.

Medical Evaluation

Apparently healthy adults of any age can increase their participation in mild and moderate physical activities without a medical examination. Mild and moderate exercise is defined as walking or other activities of a comparable intensity and usual daily activities. The exercise program recommended here simply involves, at least initially, doing more of what you are already doing. You will not be encouraged to start out with unfamiliar and vigorous activities.

Mild and moderate activities can be done with relative ease and can be sustained comfortably for a prolonged period of time, such as up to an hour. It also is important that you begin and progress slowly in your exercise program. Be alert for unusual signs or symptoms during exercise as I described earlier.

Apparently healthy, as used above, means that you have no history or evidence of major chronic diseases, such as heart disease, stroke, hypertension, diabetes, arthritis, or any other health problem that gives you concern. Be conservative, and if you believe that it is wise to contact your doctor, do so. Your doctor can then decide if there is a need for an examination.

Do I Need an Exercise Test?

Your doctor can answer this question from a medical perspective. But in addition to providing diagnostic information, an exercise test can be useful in other ways. An estimate of your physical fitness made at the outset can be used later to show progress, but it is not necessary.

In fact, my position is that exercise tests are unnecessary for most people. I am not opposed to testing, but see it as another potential barrier to changing exercise behavior. A test is simply not needed for healthy individuals who plan to make the modest lifestyle changes recommended in this book.

Later, I will show you how you can participate in a low-level walking test to get some estimate of your physical fitness level so that you can measure your own progress, if you desire.

ADDING UP THE PROS AND CONS

This chapter should have helped you think about whether you have the desire and are ready to increase your physical activity. At this point you may want to review your thoughts and see if you are ready to move toward a commitment of becoming more physically active.

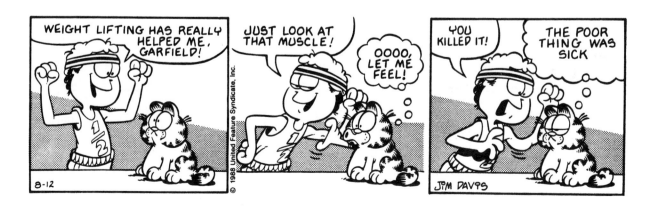

Review of Attitudes, Beliefs and Knowledge

What are your feelings about increasing your physical activity? Are you ready to make a change? Do you need more information, or do you need to wait a while to make a decision? For help in your review, please answer the following questions.

What Are My Attitudes and Beliefs About Physical Activity?

1. Do you believe that low levels of physical activity and physical fitness increase the risk of several health problems?　　YES　　NO

2. Do you think that your own health would be better if you got more exercise?　　YES　　NO

3. Do you understand the value of moderate exercise?　　YES　　NO

4. Do you think that you might feel better if you were more physically active?　　YES　　NO

5. Can you think of some physical activities that you enjoy?　　YES　　NO

A careful review of your thoughts and feelings about these questions may help you get ready to make changes in your physical activity. The quiz on the next page is designed to test your knowledge on exercise. Please answer the questions and then turn to Appendix B for the answers.

Testing Your Knowledge About Exercise

Please answer the questions below to see how well you know the effects of increased physical activity. The answers to these questions can be found in Appendix B.

True   False   1.   There is no such thing as a slow or under-active metabolism.

True   False   2.   Exercise isn't of much use for dieters because it burns relatively few calories

True   False   3.   Exercise can help prevent the loss of muscle tissue from the body.

True   False   4.   Walking one mile burns nearly the same number of calories as running the mile.

True   False   5.   Expensive exercise suits are worth the money because the special materials help the body.

True   False   6.   Climbing the stairs requires more energy per minute than traditional exercises, like swimming and jogging.

True   False   7.   Your resting pulse will increase as you lose weight and get in better condition.

True   False   8.   To get a cardiovascular training effect, there must be the right combination of frequency, intensity, and duration.

True   False   9.   No exercise can help you lose fat in specific parts of your body.

True   False   10. There are many benefits to jogging and cycling. They are good forms of exercise for people trying to lose weight.

True   False   11. Using stairs is a convenient and accessible way for many people to increase activity.

True   False   12. American adults are physically more active than they were 200 years ago.

True   False   13. You should not exercise if you feel hungry because exercise will increase your appetite.

True   False   14. When you go on a diet, your body loses fat but not muscle tissue.

True   False   15. Small, incremental, and consistent exercising activities can provide large benefits for the dieter.

CHOOSING TO CHANGE

Advantages and Disadvantages of Exercise for Me

People make decisions about changing health behavior for different reasons. I cannot know what factors might cause you to decide to increase your exercise. A couple of real life examples of what caused others to change may give you some help in deciding if the time is right for a change in your life.

CASE EXAMPLE

Lil's Picture

For the first 20 years I knew her, my wife's mother was quite sedentary. She had lived her entire life in Brooklyn where she did a little bit of walking down the block for shopping, or to the subway station. Still, for the most part, she was inactive. She had no planned exercise program, and my father-in-law did a lot of the heavy housework and yard work.

In the past couple of years, Lil has changed her exercise habits. She walks regularly and even participates in Fun Walk/Jog events at road races. What caused her to change after decades of inactivity? The answer came when someone took her picture at Easter. When she saw the photograph, her reaction was one of disbelief, "That isn't me." She suddenly realized that her dress size had crept up a couple of notches too. She decided to change. Now she is back to her old dress size, looks better, feels better, and is much happier. What will cause you to change?

The Jogging Ex-Principal

A friend of ours, a retired principal of a large urban high school, started jogging late in life. She became very serious about it. She ran every day to build up her mileage and then began to run in races. Gladys not only ran in races, but she ran to win. She was quite competitive and kept trying to improve her best times in the 10K races. I remember a letter she wrote to the editor of the newspaper after one of the biggest races in the state where she placed third among the over-50 women's group. She was very upset that the race organizers did not have a category for over-60 women, which she would have won handily. There was a category for over-60 men, and she thought there should have been one for women. The next year there was.

Gladys was asked, "Why did you start running at your age?" She replied, "My mother is in her 80s and my grandmother lived to be 96, so I figure that I have a lot of years left. If I am going to live that long, I want to be healthy and fit enough to enjoy it."

Please list on page 28, all of the advantages and disadvantages related to your plan to increase your physical activity. I will ask you to review and modify this list later because some of your reasons may change.

Under advantages, you may list such things as:

- increased energy	- improved health
- weight loss	- stress reduction

Disadvantages may include:

- **don't like to exercise**   - **do not have time**

- **I am afraid of injury**   - **I don't like the way I look in exercise clothes.**

The reasons should be your reasons, not mine. Be honest and give some careful thought to the question.

(SAMPLE)

Advantages of Becoming More Physically Active

1. *I will feel better*

2. *Other people will think of me as active*

3. *My health will improve*

4. *I will have more energy to do more things*

5. *I will like myself more*

6. *I want to be active as I get older*

Disadvantages of Becoming More Physically Active

1. *People may make fun of me*

2. *I don't have time to exercise*

3. *I don't feel good when I exercise too hard*

4. *I can't afford to buy nice exercise clothes*

5. *I'm too embarrased to go to exercise classes*

6. *Exercising doesn't sound like fun*

27

Now, please complete your own list of advantages and disadvantages:

Advantages of Becoming More Physically Active

1. _____

2. _____

3. _____

4. _____

5. _____

6. _____

Disadvantages of Becoming More Physically Active

1. _____

2. _____

3. _____

4. _____

5. _____

6. _____

It is entirely possible that your list of disadvantages may outweigh your list of advantages. That is fine. At this point, I am just asking you to consider carefully whether or not you really want to change your physical activity habits. Obviously, I hope you do. But if you do not, there is nothing to be lost by sitting comfortably and continuing to read a bit further in this book.

If the advantages win, let's see if you are ready to exercise.

Please answer the questions below to see if you are now ready to begin exercising. You may be more ready to start than you think.

Are You Ready to Exercise Quiz?

Please answer the following questions by circling YES or NO.

1.	Are you able to climb stairs?	YES	NO
2.	Can you walk a half mile without stopping?	YES	NO
3.	Do you believe that you would feel better if you increased your exercise and improved your fitness?	YES	NO
4.	Would you like to get through the day without becoming tired?	YES	NO
5.	Are you willing to budget some time for exercise?	YES	NO
6.	Do you think you will have the motivation to exercise on those days when you don't quite feel like it or when the weather is bad?	YES	NO
7.	Are you confident that you can at least make a start, and try exercise for a few weeks?	YES	NO
8.	Have you ever been physically fit, and did you like the feeling?	YES	NO
9.	Can you find someone to exercise with?	YES	NO
10.	Do you have a convenient place to exercise?	YES	NO
11.	When you think about exercise, do you develop a positive picture in your mind?	YES	NO

The more YES responses you circled, the greater the chances that you will be able to make changes successfully in your physical activity habits. If you were able to say YES to at least seven or eight of the questions, chances are good that you are ready to proceed with your exercise plan. If you only circled two or three YES responses, perhaps you should review the advantages of regular exercise.

If you still have a low level of motivation, maybe you just are not ready at the moment to make changes in your physical activity. If this is the case, do not try to make activity changes now; continue to read the following chapters and continue to examine your motivation to change.

As you have reviewed this chapter, you can see now why our high-fat, high-calorie diets and sedentary lifestyles have made it harder to stay physically fit. I have begun to show you how easy it is to moderately increase you physical activity. You can now apply this knowledge and be on your way to commiting to a more active lifestyle.

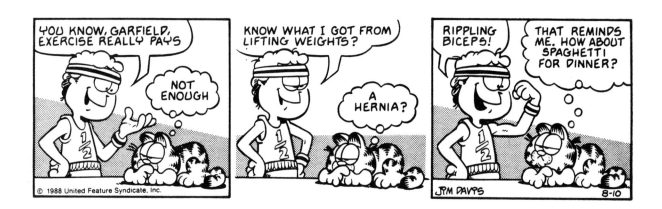

Chapter 2

BECOMING COMMITTED

You have carefully evaluated your attitudes and beliefs about exercise, and you've decided to continue to the next step. This chapter will give you more information about exercise and help you assess your current levels of physical activity and physical fitness. You can then use this information to plan your program and monitor changes in both your activity and fitness levels. You will review the pros and cons of changing your physical activity habits. Hopefully, your motivation to change will intensify and you will become committed to a new, more active lifestyle.

SELF-ASSESSMENT

In this section, you will learn how to evaluate your physical activity and physical fitness. This will involve making a few measurements, recording your activity, and some simple calculations. Don't worry - it is not difficult.

Measuring Your Physical Activity

To measure your physical activity level, you need to record or recall the type and amount of activity you did during a specified period of time. There are several ways to do this. The method presented here is relatively simple. It is a valid estimate of your total activity and provides an activity score in calories. Body weight is a major factor in the total number of calories you burn, so your score will be presented in calories per kilogram of body weight. This makes comparison to accepted standards easier and provides a stable figure for you to use to track your progress, regardless of whether you gain or lose weight.

Using METs as a Standard Measure

To estimate the amount of energy you expend, you'll use METs. MET means a metabolic equivalent, or the energy (calories) a person expends while resting quietly. A general guideline is that a person spends one calorie for each kilogram of body weight per hour. Thus, a 70-kilogram (154-pound) person burns 70 calories each hour while at rest. METs are expressed as multiples of this resting rate. Two METs, for example, means you are burning energy at double your resting rate (at about 140 calories/hour if you weigh

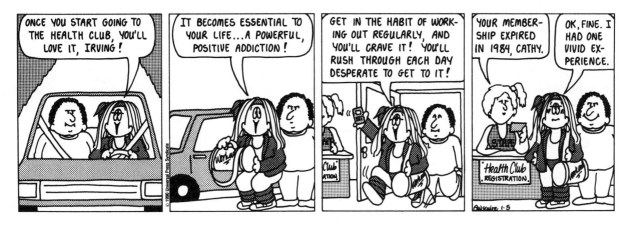

Panel 1: ONCE YOU START GOING TO THE HEALTH CLUB, YOU'LL LOVE IT, IRVING!

Panel 2: IT BECOMES ESSENTIAL TO YOUR LIFE...A POWERFUL, POSITIVE ADDICTION!

Panel 3: GET IN THE HABIT OF WORKING OUT REGULARLY, AND YOU'LL CRAVE IT! YOU'LL RUSH THROUGH EACH DAY DESPERATE TO GET TO IT!

Panel 4: YOUR MEMBERSHIP EXPIRED IN 1984, CATHY. / OK, FINE. I HAD ONE VIVID EXPERIENCE.

70 kilograms), three METs at triple the resting rate, and so forth. You will see how this simple concept can be used to keep a record of your daily energy expenditure.

To estimate your energy expenditure, you need to know how many hours you spend at various MET levels during the day and your body weight in kilograms. To convert your weight from pounds to kilograms, divide your weight in pounds by 2.2, or use the conversion table below.

Weight Conversion Table

Your Weight In Pounds	Your Weight In Kilograms	Your Weight In Pounds	Your Weight In Kilograms
100	45	180	82
105	48	185	84
110	50	190	86
115	52	195	88
120	54	200	91
125	57	205	93
130	59	210	95
135	61	215	98
140	64	220	100
145	66	225	102
150	68	230	104
155	70	235	107
160	73	240	109
165	75	245	111
170	77	250	113
175	79	255	116

If your weight falls between the five-pound increments, you can round to the nearest kilogram. If your weight is more or less than shown in the table, you can calculate your weight in kilograms by dividing your weight in pounds by 2.2.

Physical Activity and METs

You can estimate the number of calories you expend daily if you know the number of hours you spend in activities at the various MET levels. To simplify this process, we will group activities with similar energy costs into categories.

Most people spend the greatest part of the day in light activities. It would be difficult to remember or record everything that you did in this category. Fortunately, you do not have to record activities in that detail. If the other categories are accurately recorded, the time spent in light activities can be obtained by subtraction. On the next page are some guidelines to help you record your daily activities in the proper category.

- **Sleep [1 MET]** -- This category is self-explanatory. You simply record the number of hours you sleep (at night and in naps) during a 24-hour period.

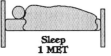
Sleep
1 MET

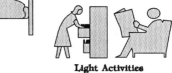
Light Activities
1 to 3 METs

- **Light activities [1-3 METs]** -- This will be obtained by subtraction later. Most of your daily activities, such as desk work or standing, will fall into this category.

- **Moderate activities [3-5 METs]** -- This category includes all activities that require 3 to 5 times resting energy expenditure. One example of this type of activity is walking. Walking at 3 mph (20 minutes per mile) requires 3 METs, and walking at 4 mph (15 minutes per mile) requires 4 METs. Most adults can walk comfortably at 3 to 4 mph and that speed is usually described as a brisk pace. It is not race walking or a casual stroll; it is the pace that you might move if you were in a bit of a hurry to make an appointment. Even sedentary and unfit individuals can walk at this speed for several minutes without undue fatigue.

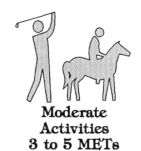
Moderate
Activities
3 to 5 METs

- **Hard activities [5-7 METs]** -- Hard activities are more strenuous that brisk walking, but not as strenuous as running. A good example is doubles tennis. There is a problem, however, in classifying sports activities. Tournament doubles tennis may belong in the very hard category. On the other hand, it is possible to play doubles tennis and scarcely move around at all. In this latter case, doubles might even belong in the light activity category. So for sports, household, occupational, and recreational activities that can be performed at different paces, you have to use some judgment as to where they should be placed. Again, I refer you back to the walking example. If a recreational activity seems to be about the same intensity as brisk walking, classify it as moderate. If it is more or less strenuous, classify it accordingly.

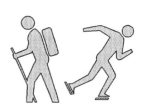
Hard
Activities
5 to 7 METs

- **Very hard activities [8+ METs]** -- Activities in this group are quite strenuous for most people. Sedentary and unfit individuals cannot sustain very hard activities for more than a few minutes without becoming fatigued. Running at any speed qualifies for this category. Vigorous sports involving a lot of running, such as soccer or basketball, are usually very hard activities. If you are trying to classify an activity, ask yourself if it is as hard as running. If the answer is no, then assign the activity to a lower intensity category.

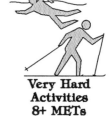
Very Hard
Activities
8+ METs

Appendix A, on page 111, gives a more complete list of the MET value of different activities. If an activity you performed is not on the list, mentally compare its intensity to that of brisk walking. If the activity seems less strenuous than walking, it probably belongs in the light category. If it is more strenuous, it should be assigned to the hard or even the very hard category.

There are several other tips to remember when you are assigning activities to categories and recording the time for each activity category.

First, it is important to remember that you probably spend most of your time in light activity. Many unpleasant and boring household or occupational tasks may leave you feeling tired, but their energy expenditure is not great, and they belong in the light category. A store clerk, for example, might spend most of the day standing and feel tired. The energy cost, however, would be small.

It is also important to record only the actual time you were physically doing the activity. You might spend three hours at the beach, but only 30 minutes swimming. You should only record the 30 minutes (in either the hard or very hard category, depending on the speed) you actually swam in this category. Remember, you do not have to record the time spent in rest breaks, time out for meals, or other light activities. This time will be derived by subtraction.

Remember, too, that the rate at which many activities are performed makes a large difference in the actual energy cost. Digging in the garden, for example, is generally a very hard activity, but it is possible to dig very slowly and make it a moderate activity.

Activities that are broken up by interruptions can present a problem. Take weight lifting, for example. Suppose you spend 30 minutes weight lifting. Some of the time is spent lifting; some is spent moving to the next station, adding weights, and preparing to lift. If you record only the time actually spent lifting, it would go into the very hard category. If you record the entire 30 minutes, place it in the moderate category.

Be consistent over time in the judgments you make about where to place activities and how you record your time. This will enable you to be accurate over time so that you can measure your progress with more precision.

It is difficult to recall short bouts of exercise, yet building activities such as stair climbing into your routine can have a significant impact on your overall energy expenditure. For the purposes of the physical activity score, I suggest that you not try to keep track of exercise bouts of less than two minutes. At the end of the day you can sum the short (two minutes or more) bouts. For example, if you took six two-minute walks, add 12 minutes to the moderate activity category. Stair climbing can make an important contribution to your physical activity score. A flight only takes a few seconds to climb, so if you climb several flights in a day, figure out the total time spent climbing, and add it to the very hard category. Be careful not to overestimate the amount of time spent climbing.

CASE EXAMPLE

Pam's Example

Pam is a CPA and has a sedentary job. During the busy season, Pam has very little time for scheduled physical activity. She lives in an apartment and does not do any yard or garden work. She also hires a cleaning service and does not have to do any heavy housework. Pam was concerned about her physical fitness, so she joined an exercise class and does some walking on her lunch break.

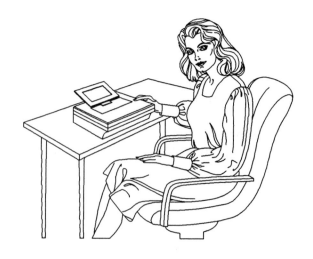

Here is what she did yesterday. After 7 hours of sleep, she dressed, had breakfast, and went to work. She took the bus, which required a five-minute walk from her apartment to the bus stop, and a 10-minute walk from where she leaves the bus to her office. She worked all day at her desk, doing little moving around the office. At lunch time, she took a 30-minute walk to view a new outdoor sculpture at city hall. After work, she participated in a one-hour aerobics class at the YWCA across the street from her office. She then took the bus home, prepared and ate her dinner, read for a while, and went to bed.

The Energy Expenditure Chart

To help you calculate your daily energy expenditure, I have developed a simple energy expenditure chart. A blank chart can be found on page 37. Feel free to make copies of this chart for your own personal use. Working through an example should convince you that this is not a difficult task, and the information it will provide you will be well worth the effort.

Today's Date _June 1, 1991_

(Pam's Sample)
Energy Expenditure Chart

	(1) Activity Type	(2) METs	X	(3) Hours of Activity	=	(4) Calorie Expenditure per kg of Weight
1.	Sleep	1		7		7
2.	Moderate	4		1		4
3.	Hard	6		1		6
4.	Very Hard	10		0		0
5.	Total hours from 1-4			9		
6.	Light*	1.5		15		22.5
7.	Total calories expended per kg today					39.5
8.	Weight (in kg)					54
9.	Total calories expended					2,133

*This number is derived by subtracting the total on line 5 from 24.

Let's now review Pam's day of activity and work through a sample energy expenditure chart.

LINE 1 - First, Pam spent seven hours sleeping. Line one of the chart is for sleeping and has a MET value of one. In column three, on line one, we will record the seven hours Pam spent sleeping.

LINE 2 - Pam also spent a total of one hour walking (30 minutes in conjunction with her bus rides and 30 minutes during lunch). Since her walking was a brisk walk, this activity falls into the moderate category. On line two we will record one hour in column three. In the sample chart, I use an average of four METs for moderate activity.

LINE 3 - Pam's exercise class is harder than walking, but not as hard as running. Therefore, the one-hour class would be recorded in the hard activity category on line three. An average of six METs is used for this category.

LINE 4 - Pam did not do any physical activities that would be classified as very hard. In column three on line four, we would record zero.

LINE 5 - In column three of line five, we will total the number of hours recorded in lines one through four. We do this so that we can derive the number of light activity hours. In Pam's example, the total of lines one through four is equal to nine.

LINE 6 - The number of light activity hours is derived by subtracting the number on line five from 24. Pam spent a total of nine hours in non-light activities, thus the number of hours she spent on light activities is 15 (the difference between 24 and nine). We use 1.5 METs for this level of activity.

LINE 7 - We multiply the number of hours spent in each activity category (column three) by the number of METs assigned to each category (column two) and record the product in column four. On line seven, we sum the numbers in column four (lines 1-6). This number is the total number of calories Pam expended for the day per each kg of weight.

LINE 8 - On this line, we record Pam's weight. Remember, weight needs to be in kilograms (kg). Refer back to the table on page 32 if you need help with the conversion.

LINE 9 - We multiply the daily calories expended per kg (line seven) by weight (line eight) and enter the product on line nine. This gives the total calories expended during the day through physical activity. In Pam's example, she expended a total of 2,133 calories during the day.

You should keep in mind that these are estimates. There are other factors that go into determining energy expenditure, and there is some variability between individuals. The same can be said about estimating the number of calories you take in. Both procedures are valid; accuracy is increased if you use the same techniques over time and are consistent in the judgments you make about categorizing activities.

To put your energy expenditure in perspective, consider these examples:

The person who stays in bed all day has a score of 24.

The person who does not do any moderate, hard or very hard activity has a score of 32.

The person who does two hours of moderate activity (household work, some walking, etc.), one hour of hard yard work, and one hour of running, has a score of 50.

Keeping a Record

I suggest that you keep a record of your physical activities, calculate the daily energy expenditure, and plot the results on a graph similar to the one on page 38. You may want to make copies of the graph for use in the future. Keeping a record of your activity can help you make changes and stay with your new routine. It may be helpful to keep the graph in a prominent place, such as on your refrigerator door or on a bulletin board by your telephone, so that you are reminded on a regular basis.

You should begin calculating your energy expenditure now and graphing the results, even though you are not starting to change your physical activity. Keeping the record for several days will give you practice in doing the record-keeping and calculations and will provide a more accurate and stable baseline of your current activity. A good estimate of your current activity is important so that small increments of progress can be seen when you begin to make changes.

Name _____   Today's Date _____

Energy Expenditure Chart

	(1) Activity Type	(2) METs	X	(3) Hours of Activity	=	(4) Calorie Expenditure per kg of Weight
1.	Sleep	1		_____		_____
2.	Moderate	4		_____		_____
3.	Hard	6		_____		_____
4.	Very Hard	10		_____		_____
5.	Total hours from 1-4			_____		
6.	Light*	1.5		_____		_____
7.	Total calories expended per kg today					_____
8.	Weight (in kg)					_____
9.	Total calories expended					_____

*This number is derived by subtracting the total on line 5 from 24.

Directions for completing The Energy Expenditure Chart

- **Keep a record of your daily activities.**

- **At the end of the day, calculate how many hours you spent in each level of activity.**

- **Put your totals in the appropriate blanks on the chart above.**

- **The total in line number 7 is the number you will place on the your Calorie Expenditure Graph on page 38.**

- **If you multiply your total in line 7 with your body weight (in kg), you will have your total caloric expenditure for the day.**

Please refer back to Pam's example calculations if you need help with The Energy Expenditure Chart.

Caloric Expenditure

(Sample)

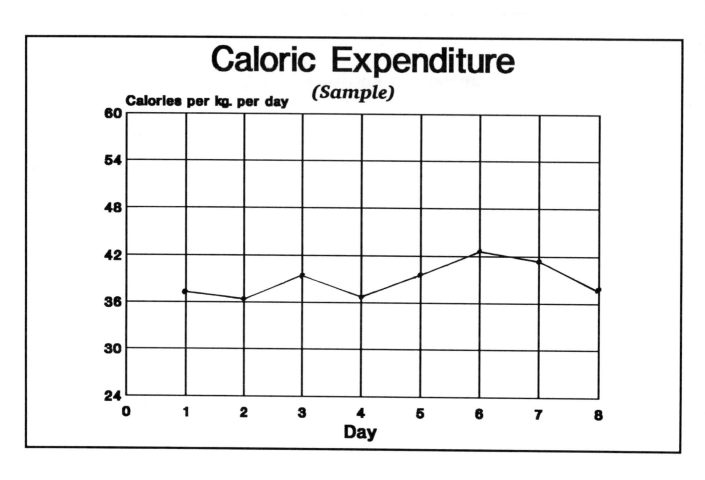

Caloric Expenditure

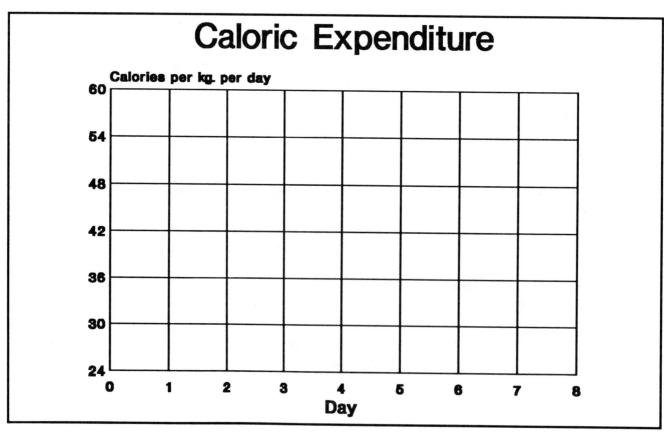

TESTING YOUR PHYSICAL FITNESS

It is more important to have a good record of your physical activity than it is to know your physical fitness. The emphasis here is on measuring and recording your daily energy expenditure, not physical fitness. However, many of you may still want to have some estimate of your physical fitness level. As I mentioned in the introduction, there are many different types of fitness. To avoid possible confusion, I will be referring here to aerobic fitness, sometimes referred to as cardiovascular fitness. This is the type of fitness that is related to the risk of several chronic diseases and death.

Testing Aerobic Fitness

Aerobic fitness can be measured quite accurately in a laboratory, using a treadmill or stationary cycle. Fitness can be evaluated by an exercise test as part of a medical examination, although, as stated earlier, most people do not need an exercise test prior to beginning a mild or moderate exercise program. Low-level fitness tests sometimes are given by health clubs, YMCAs, and YWCAs or in a worksite health promotion program. If you have access to such a service, you can have an exercise professional evaluate your fitness level.

You can also estimate your own fitness level with a simple, self-administered walking test that was developed at the Institute for Aerobics Research in Dallas. It offers you an opportunity to evaluate your aerobic fitness. It is safe and not too strenuous. Prior to taking this, or any other self-administered fitness test, you should complete the "Physical Activity Readiness Questionnaire," presented in the previous chapter.

Also familiarize yourself with the "When to Stop Exercise" section of Chapter 1 on page 20. Do not take the fitness test if you have any "YES" responses on the "Physical Activity Readiness Questionnaire" (pages 21 & 22), and stop the test if problem symptoms arise during the course of taking the test.

Tips and Precautions for Performing Fitness Assessments

The following tips and suggestions should help prepare you for a physical fitness assessment:

- If you experience unusual pain or discomfort during any part of the test, **STOP IMMEDIATELY** and consult your physician.

- Wait one or two hours after your last meal before performing the assessments.

- Wear comfortable, loose-fitting clothing and comfortable, well-padded shoes suitable for walking. Perform a few warm-up exercises before starting the fitness assessments.

- If you do the tests outdoors in a hot climate, test during the cooler hours of the morning or evening to avoid the heat. Do not take the tests outdoors on days that are extremely cold or windy.

- If possible, have a friend or family member help you with the tests. It's easy and fun to conduct the tests in a group.

- Practice taking your pulse before taking the walking test. The following section should help you do this.

TAKING YOUR PULSE

In most people, the pulse can be felt wherever a large artery lies near the surface--at the neck, temple, or wrist. The pulse can also be felt on the chest near the heart. To take your pulse at the neck, temple, or wrist, place your first two fingers gently over the artery. Use your palm if taking the pulse on the chest over the heart. Then count the number of times you feel your heart beat in 15 seconds and multiply by 4. This gives the number of beats per minute. If you're taking an exercising pulse rate, begin counting immediately after stopping the exercise. Your pulse rate drops rapidly after stopping exercise, and if you wait even a few seconds, it will slow and you will underestimate your exercising pulse rate. Move around a bit while taking your post-exercise pulse rate to avoid having your blood "pool" in your legs, which can cause lightheadness or fainting. Practice taking your pulse until you feel confident and can find it quickly.

Many people find it helpful to use the 15-second pulse count instead of the per-minute pulse count. I have included the following pulse rate table to help make the arithmetic a little easier.

Pulse Rate Table

15 second pulse count	Pulse rate in beats per minute	15 second pulse count	Pulse rate in beats per minute
25	100	36	144
26	104	37	148
27	108	38	152
28	112	39	156
29	116	40	160
30	120	41	164
31	124	42	168
32	128	43	172
33	132	44	176
34	136	45	180
35	140	46	184

The Institute for Aerobics Research One-Mile Walking Test
(reprinted with permission)

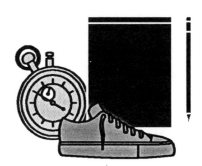

Purpose

To measure the ability of the heart and lungs to take in and deliver oxygen to the body during exercise.

Equipment Needed

- Stopwatch or watch with a second hand
- Pencil and paper to record time and pulse rate
- Comfortable walking shoes.

Special Considerations

- Don't drink caffeinated beverages for at least three hours before the test. Caffeine elevates the pulse rate and would affect the validity of the test.

- If you're taking blood pressure or other medication that prevents the heart rate from increasing during exercise or causes it to increase higher than normal, this test would be invalid for you. Don't take this test if you're currently using any of these types of medications:

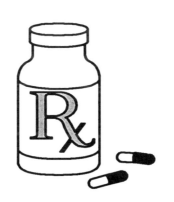

Alpha blockers

Beta blockers

Calcium channel blockers

Nitrates

Combined alpha and
beta blockers

Centrally acting
adrenergic inhibitors

Non-adrenergic
peripheral vasodilators

Peripheral acting
adrenergic inhibitors

Bronchodilators

Cold medications

Tricyclic antidepressants

Major tranquilizers

Diet medications

Thyroid medications

Procedures

1. Find a smooth, level surface where you can accurately measure a one-mile distance: a track at a school, a measured walking course in a park, a shopping mall, or even your neighborhood streets. If you plan to walk on the street, avoid stoplights and heavy traffic areas.

2. Warm up for several minutes by stretching or walking briskly.

3. Walk (do not run) one mile as quickly as you can without straining. Maintain a constant pace.

4. After you finish the one-mile walk, observe the time and keep moving slowly while immediately taking your pulse for 15 seconds. Convert your 15-second pulse rate to beats per minute by multiplying by 4, or use the conversion chart on page 40. For example, if your 15-second pulse count is 32 beats, your pulse rate is 128 beats per minute. Record your one-minute pulse rate.

5. Record the time it took to walk the one-mile distance in **minutes** and **seconds**. Most people take between 10 and 20 minutes to walk one mile.

6. Continue to walk slowly for a few minutes to allow your heart rate and blood pressure to return to normal levels.

7. Use the charts on pages 42 & 43 and the directions on page 44 to determine your current aerobic fitness level.

Men
Assumes a body weight of 175 pounds

Age	Heart Rate	Low Fitness	Moderate Fitness	High Fitness
20-29	110	>19:36	17:06 - 19:36	<17:06
	120	>19:10	16:36 - 19:10	<16:36
	130	>18:35	16:06 - 18:35	<16:06
	140	>18:06	15:36 - 18:06	<15:36
	150	>17:36	15:10 - 17:36	<15:10
	160	>17:09	14:42 - 17:09	<14:42
	170	>16:39	14:12 - 16:39	<14:12
30-39	110	>18:21	15:54 - 18:21	<15:54
	120	>17:52	15:24 - 17:52	<15:24
	130	>17:22	14:54 - 17:22	<14:54
	140	>16:54	14:30 - 16:54	<14:30
	150	>16:26	14:00 - 16:26	<14:00
	160	>15:58	13:30 - 15:58	<13:30
	170	>15:28	13:01 - 15:28	<13:01
40-49	110	>18:05	15:38 - 18:05	<15:38
	120	>17:36	15:09 - 17:36	<15:09
	130	>17:07	14:41 - 17:07	<14:41
	140	>16:38	14:12 - 16:38	<14:12
	150	>16:09	13:42 - 16:09	<13:42
	160	>15:42	13:15 - 15:42	<13:15
	170	>15:12	12:45 - 15:12	<12:45
50-59	110	>17:49	15:22 - 17:49	<15:22
	120	>17:20	14:53 - 17:20	<14:53
	130	>16:51	14:24 - 16:51	<14:24
	140	>16:22	13:51 - 16:22	<13:51
	150	>15:53	13:26 - 15:53	<13:26
	160	>15:26	12:59 - 15:26	<12:59
	170	>14:56	12:30 - 14:56	<12:30
60+	110	>17:55	15:33 - 17:55	<15:33
	120	>17:24	15:04 - 17:24	<15:04
	130	>16:57	14:36 - 16:57	<14:36
	140	>16:28	14:07 - 16:28	<14:07
	150	>15:59	13:39 - 15:59	<13:39
	160	>15:30	13:10 - 15:30	<13:10
	170	>15:04	12:42 - 15:04	<12:42

For every 10 lbs. over 175 lbs., men must walk 15 seconds faster to qualify for a fitness category.

For every 10 lbs. under 175 lbs., men can walk 15 seconds slower to qualify for a fitness category.

Women

Assumes a body weight of 125 pounds

Age	Heart Rate	Low Fitness	Moderate Fitness	High Fitness
20-29	110	>20:57	19:08 - 20:57	<19:08
	120	>20:27	18:38 - 20:27	<18:38
	130	>20:00	18:12 - 20:00	<18:12
	140	>19:30	17:42 - 19:30	<17:42
	150	>19:00	17:12 - 19:00	<17:12
	160	>18:30	16:42 - 18:30	<16:42
	170	>18:00	16:12 - 18:00	<16:12
30-39	110	>19:46	17:52 - 19:46	<17:52
	120	>19:18	17:24 - 19:18	<17:24
	130	>18:48	16:54 - 18:48	<16:54
	140	>18:18	16:24 - 18:18	<16:24
	150	>17:48	15:54 - 17:48	<15:54
	160	>17:18	15:24 - 17:18	<15:24
	170	>16:54	14:55 - 16:54	<14:55
40-49	110	>19:15	17:20 - 19:15	<17:20
	120	>18:45	16:50 - 18:45	<16:50
	130	>18:18	16:24 - 18:18	<16:24
	140	>17:48	15:54 - 17:48	<15:54
	150	>17:18	15:24 - 17:18	<15:24
	160	>16:48	14:54 - 16:48	<14:54
	170	>16:18	14:25 - 16:18	<14:25
50-59	110	>18:40	17:04 - 18:40	<17:04
	120	>18:12	16:36 - 18:12	<16:36
	130	>17:42	16:06 - 17:42	<16:06
	140	>17:18	15:36 - 17:18	<15:36
	150	>16:48	15:06 - 16:48	<15:06
	160	>16:18	14:36 - 16:18	<14:36
	170	>15:48	14:06 - 15:48	<14:06
60+	110	>18:00	16:36 - 18:00	<16:36
	120	>17:30	16:06 - 17:30	<16:06
	130	>17:01	15:37 - 17:01	<15:37
	140	>16:31	15:09 - 16:31	<15:09
	150	>16:02	14:39 - 16:02	<14:39
	160	>15:32	14:12 - 15:32	<14:12
	170	>15:04	13:42 - 15:04	<13:42

For every 10 lbs. over 125 lbs., women must walk 15 seconds faster to qualify for a fitness category.

For every 10 lbs. under 125 lbs., women can walk 15 seconds slower to qualify for a fitness category.

Directions

On the left side of the previous charts (be sure that you are using the correct chart for your sex), find your age category and pulse rate. If your exact pulse rate isn't shown, round it off to the nearest 10 beats. To the right of this value are the one-mile walk times for "Low," "Moderate," and "High" fitness levels. You may need to make an adjustment as noted at the bottom of the charts, if your weight differs from the specified weight.

Note that for a given heart rate, the older you are, the faster you must walk to qualify for a fitness category. This is because a person's greatest possible heart rate decreases with age. Therefore, for any given heart rate, a younger person is working at a relatively lower percentage of maximum aerobic power (hence he or she is more physically fit) than an older person.

The following example will help you understand the scoring and classification of your fitness level. Suppose that Janet is 46 years old and weighs 145 pounds. She walks one mile in 17:15 (17 minutes and 15 seconds), and her heart rate at the end of the walk was 143 beats per minute. First, because she is 20 pounds over the 125 pounds specified in the footnote in the women's table, she must add 30 seconds to her time (15 seconds for every 10 pounds over 125 pounds). Thus, her adjusted time to be used in the scoring is 17:45.

Next, she would find her appropriate age category on the women's chart. Her heart rate was 143 beats per minute, so she should find the line closest to that number, which is the line for 140 beats per minute. She can see that her adjusted time of 17:45 falls within the moderate fitness category (time range of 15:54 - 17:48). Note that she just made it into the moderate category with only 3 seconds to spare. She might decide that is too close to the low category, and may wish to improve her fitness.

When interpreting your test results, remember that the test provides **an estimate** of your aerobic fitness level. More precise values can be obtained by a professional in a testing laboratory, but the walking test is accurate for general purposes. The test described above can give you an idea of your relative fitness level. You can also use it to monitor changes in fitness level as you increase your exercise behavior.

A Simple Walking Test

Fitness improvement can be checked even more simply. This approach involves two steps:

- Walk any course that takes you 4-6 minutes to complete. It does not have to be flat, and you do not need to know the distance. You do not have to walk it fast or at any particular speed.

- Time how long it takes you to cover the course to the nearest second. Take your heart rate for 15 seconds immediately after finishing the walk, and multiply by four to get beats per minute. Record both how long it took you to complete the walk and your heart rate. This is your starting point.

As you gradually increase your physical activity, your aerobic fitness will improve. Your muscles will improve their ability to use oxygen and release energy to perform the work. Your heart will become stronger and able to pump more blood with each beat. This will cause your resting heart rate to go down and will lower your heart rate for a standard exercise task.

Therefore, after a few weeks, if you repeat the simple test described above, you should note changes. Your time for the walk around the same course should be less, your heart rate should be lower immediately after the walk, or both responses may change.

CASE EXAMPLE

Patty and the Monument

Boston is a wonderful city to visit. A few years ago, my family was on vacation there with some friends. We had a great time. We did some sightseeing, visited the Kennedy Museum, attended a play, ate good seafood, and soaked up the local color. One afternoon, we visited the Bunker Hill Monument. It is an impressive structure that is open to the public, and is maintained by the National Park Service. Everyone wanted to climb to the top to enjoy the view. Our friend Patty, who was about 35 years old at the time, tried, but she couldn't make it to the top. She was simply too unfit. Breathing heavily, she went back down and waited for us. The photo taken at the top includes everyone in the group, except Patty.

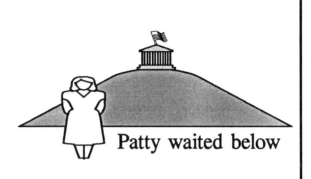

Patty waited below

I don't know if the monument adventure is the reason, but Patty is now exercising, has lost weight, and can enjoy more active leisure time activities. Do you want to be like Patty, left out of activities because you are unfit? If you find that your level of fitness is limiting what you can do, or what you might like to do, you may want to make some changes in your lifestyle too.

Acceptable Standards for Physical Activity and Aerobic Fitness

In earlier sections, I reviewed the relationship between physical activity and physical fitness to health. You may remember that there is a general linear relationship, with less active and fit people being at higher risk for disease and early death. I tried to communicate the concept that moderate levels of activity and fitness are better than very low levels, and that higher levels may provide some further benefit.

Many people can benefit from increasing their activity and improving their fitness. You may want to know whether you are in the lowest fitness category or have managed to exercise enough to be in the moderate fitness category. How concerned are you about your present status? The results of the evaluations described earlier in this chapter can help answer those questions.

Physical Activity Standard

To determine where you stand, you should complete records of your physical activity for several days - a week's worth or information would be useful - and graph your daily caloric expenditure on the chart provided earlier on page 38. What is your typical score?

Score	Description
32-35	Too Sedentary
36-38	Relatively Sedentary
39-42	Moderate Activity
42+	Very Active Lifestyle

If you consistently score in the range of 32 to 35 calories per kilogram, you are probably too sedentary. Your health and function will benefit from an increase in physical activity.

Scores in the range of 36 to 38 are better, but still too low. You are leading a relatively sedentary life if your scores are in this range. You are not starting at the bottom, but a few changes to increase your activity level will place you in a much more favorable position.

If you consistently score in the range of 39 to 42 calories per kilogram, you are probably in the moderate fitness group shown on the mortality charts in Chapter 1. You are exercising enough to obtain important health and functional benefits. Keep up the good work. You can still improve; and if you do, you can expect a further reduction in health risks.

Finally, scores of 43 calories per kilogram or more are indicative of a very active lifestyle. If you have recorded and calculated accurately, you are as active as you need to be for optimal health. If you question that conclusion and think that you are not active enough, it may be that you have not accurately estimated your energy expenditure. You may want to recheck your figures. But if your figures are correct and you still want to increase your activity, that is fine. I do not believe you are likely to get much more in the way of health benefits, but you can improve your physical fitness.

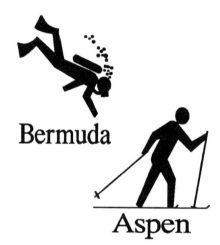

Bermuda

Aspen

I have been running 35 to 50 miles a week for nearly 20 years, so my daily energy expenditure is typically in the upper 40s in calories per kilogram per day. I recognize that this is more exercise than I need to stay healthy, but I intend to continue at this level. For me, and many others, there are additional benefits to being very active. In my case, I have a weight problem; I can keep it at least partly under control with my running. I also like the high level of fitness produced by daily running. I want to be fit enough to enjoy a few hours of snorkeling if I go to Bermuda or a few hours of cross-country skiing when I go to Aspen. I want to be fit enough to enjoy vigorous recreational activities with my family and friends, and not be left out, as Patty was in the earlier case example. Also, my daily run is an excellent "time out" period. I like to run at noon. This breaks up my day and seems to give me a fresh outlook for my afternoon's work.

You may or may not decide that a very vigorous lifestyle is for you, and that is entirely your choice. I do not presume that my choices are ideal for everyone. I am certain, however, that you will gain considerable health and functional benefits if you become active enough to get out of the very sedentary categories.

Physical Fitness Standard

Your score on the walking test can be used to evaluate your aerobic fitness level. The low fitness level corresponds to the low fitness category in the Aerobics Center Longitudinal Study described in Chapter 1. This level of fitness was associated with a greatly increased risk of early death, as shown in the figures in Chapter 1. Thus, you have a lot to lose if you are in the low fitness category on the walking test, and you should try to become more active and improve your fitness level to at least the moderate category.

If your score on the walking test was in the moderate category, your fitness is equal to the moderate category in the Aerobics Center Longitudinal Study. Your risk of early death is much less than if you were in the low fitness category, but you can lower your risk even more with just a little more exercise and further improvement in your physical fitness.

If your score on the walking test was in the high fitness category, congratulations. You are physically fit, and you have a relatively low risk of developing several chronic diseases.

Other Fitness Tests

Other types of physical fitness are important for optimal function and avoidance of disability, and may be related to some health problems. There is not a great deal of good research on the relevance, importance, and precise contributions of such things as muscular strength, muscular endurance, and flexibility on good health and the ability to function. But it does seem logical that minimal levels of these characteristics are needed. New research is underway in our program and elsewhere to address these important issues; but for the present, I am willing to assume that we should give some attention to these other types of fitness.

Our modern daily existence, at least for most of us, does not require large amounts of strength and endurance. Most of us develop adequate levels of these characteristics while we are young and active, and have more than enough to meet demands. We also seem to lose these characteristics more slowly than we lose aerobic fitness; so in the younger, and on into the middle years, low levels of strength, endurance, and flexibility are not a problem. At some point, however, the decline in these abilities begin to impinge on daily activities. For example, some of you may have noticed that it has become more difficult to tie your shoes or button your shirt. You may no longer be able to carry a couple of bags of groceries in from the car with ease. Or you may notice that other routine tasks that you used to do with no problem have become difficult or impossible. This loss of function is a gradual process and passes unnoticed until it reaches a critical level. Community surveys show that the percentage of people who need assistance with tasks, such as housework, climbing stairs, walking, or using the toilet increases dramatically in the later years. For men and women in their 80s, one-fourth to one-third need assistance with activities of daily living.

Some of this relative disability with aging is due to chronic disease. People who have had a heart attack, stroke, or some other serious health problem frequently suffer a loss of function. My hypothesis is that some, and perhaps a lot, of the decline in functional capability can be attributed to the low levels of musculoskeletal fitness - which has to do with muscle strength and endurance and joint flexibility - brought about by decades of sedentary living. Therefore, I recommend that you build and maintain a higher level of this type of fitness earlier in life, so that you can continue to function at a higher level when you are older.

I find that my parents and other older people do not fear death as much as they fear a loss of independence. "I don't want to have to go into a nursing home" is a common plea. I agree. I hope that I run out of life before I run out of the strength, endurance, and flexibility to walk and take care of myself.

Tests Of Musculoskeletal Fitness

As with aerobic fitness, the physical activity behavior to develop and maintain fitness is more important than testing these variables. But there are some simple tests you can do to evaluate musculoskeletal function.

- **Curl-ups**--Strength and endurance of the muscles of the abdominal wall can be evaluated by the curl-up test. To perform the test, lie on your back with your feet flat on the floor and you knees at about a 90° angle . The position of your hands is not particularly important, but repeat the position each time you test yourself. You may place your hands behind your head, arms across your chest, or arms by your sides. It will be more difficult to do the curl-up with your hands behind your head, and easiest with your arms by your sides. The test is done by slowly curling your upper body into a sitting position. You should raise your head first, then your shoulders, and finally come to the full sitting position. I do not know for certain how many curl-ups you should be able to do to demonstrate adequate strength and endurance of this muscle group. I do not think it is necessary to do a timed test to see how many you can do in one or two minutes; I believe that the standards for this test proposed by others, which require a few dozen curl-ups in a minute, are excessive. If you cannot do at least three to five of the curl-ups, you probably need to do some exercises to strengthen these muscles. An excellent exercise is to simply practice the test.

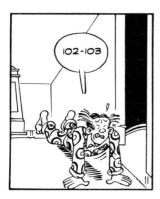 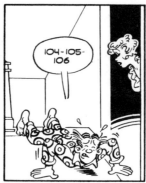 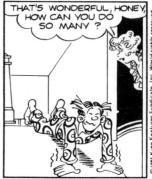 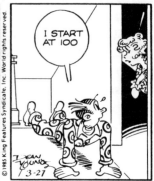

- **Push-ups**—The old push-up exercise is an excellent test of the strength of the muscles in your arms and shoulders. To perform the test, lie on the floor face down with your hands beside your shoulders. Keep your body in a straight line and use your arms to push your shoulders up until you arms are straight. If you cannot perform a push-up in this way, keep your knees on the floor and raise your body from the knees up. This will be much easier than raising your body from your toes. Once again, it is not well established how many push-ups are required for optimal function, but a good target is half a dozen of the full push-ups.

There are many other ways to improve muscle strength and endurance. You can follow a formal weight training program using weights or weight machines; you can do calisthenic exercises, such as push-ups, pull-ups, or some other activity for other muscle groups; or you can perform any other activity that causes you to exert your muscles. It doesn't matter what you do, as long as you are stressing the muscles a bit by doing more strenuous activity than you typically do.

Unfortunately, many people have the idea that weight training is a very complicated process that requires you to follow a rigid schedule and do very carefully prescribed exercises. This may be true for athletes in training or for others who are trying to get maximum muscular development. But this level of detail in unnecessary for most of us. Our objective should be to simply develop and maintain an adequate level of strength and endurance to carry out daily tasks. So look for opportunities to use your muscles at work and around home. Do some digging in the garden, some lifting, do a few calisthenics, or work a little harder than usual.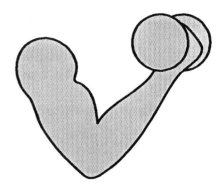

- **Flexibility tests**—It is important to maintain adequate flexibility, especially as we get older. Lack of flexibility is probably not related to any serious disease, but it can cause you to have difficulty moving. You may feel stiff or have difficulty bending or straightening. You may find it hard to get out of a chair or car.

Here are a couple of simple tests of your flexibility. You can test the flexibility of the muscles of your back and the back of your legs with the sit and reach test. To perform this test, sit on the floor with your legs straight out in front of you. Slowly stretch forward to see if you can touch your toes. Do not bounce, but stretch slowly, and repeat the movement three or four times. You should be able to touch, or at least, nearly touch your toes. If you cannot, perhaps you should do a few flexibility exercises. Repeating the sit and reach test regularly can improve flexibility in the back and legs.

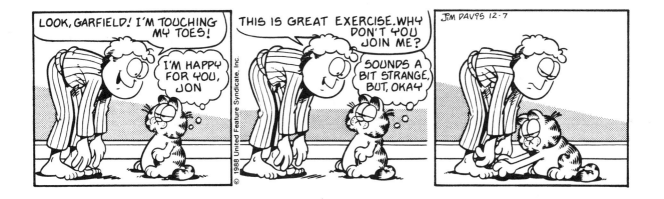

Any exercises or movements that require you to extend the range of motion around a joint can increase your flexibility. Just remember to move slowly, don't bounce, stretch your muscles, and hold the stretched position for several seconds. Repeat the exercises a few times, and do these activities several times a week. This will help you develop and maintain adequate flexibility. You do not need an elaborate professionally designed stretching program. You can probably tell which of your joints are limited in their range of motion. What tasks do you have trouble doing that you used to be able to do with ease? Consider if lack of flexibility might be a cause. Then, work out a method to stretch the joints and muscles that are affected.

Here is a simple flexibility test of the arms and shoulders. Stretch one hand behind your neck, turn the other arm with your palm facing outward, and reach between your shoulder blades. Try to touch the fingers of your hands. How close can you come? If your fingers are several inches apart, you would probably benefit from doing some flexibility exercises. You can monitor your progress in improving your flexibility by having a partner use a ruler and measure how far you can reach in the two tests described above. As your flexibility improves, the distance will decrease.

Professional Evaluation

Do you need to go to a medical clinic, an exercise club, or an exercise physiologist to get a fitness evaluation? I am not opposed to people obtaining this kind professional evaluation and advice. I have been involved in such activities for over 20 years. I directed an exercise physiology laboratory early in my career and have implemented many worksite health promotion programs in which fitness evaluations were offered. I also have helped train and certify health professionals to offer these services. Fortunately, we now have a large group of well-trained exercise professionals distributed around the country. You can obtain a detailed and objective evaluation of your fitness from them.

In recent years, I have come to realize that what I have called the "clinical approach" to exercise programming is not the complete answer. This approach calls for clients to come to the exercise professional for evaluation and instruction. There are advantages to this model. For some, being tested and receiving an exercise prescription from a professional may provide motivation. People with health problems or physical limitations may need special programs designed for them.

But there also are problems with the "clinical approach." It creates a mind-set that physical activity is an unusual and complicated human behavior. I do not agree. As I mentioned earlier, we evolved to be active animals. Physical activity is a normal and natural part of our life. We do not need very much medical and scientific instruction before going for a walk, climbing stairs, doing household and garden chores, or carrying in our groceries. Sometimes, insisting on professional testing and prescription introduces barriers to the behavioral change process. It takes time and money to obtain professional services, and this serves as a convenient excuse not to begin, for some people. There are tens of millions of sedentary and unfit adults in the U.S., and most of them do not need to see a health professional before taking a walk and generally increasing their physical activity level.

I think that you can listen to your body and direct you own program. You can do some self-testing to monitor your fitness improvement. If you have access to a fitness testing program at the YMCA or YWCA, a health club, or at your worksite, and if you would like a professional evaluation, do it. But you are capable of increasing your activity and monitoring your progress without it.

ARE YOU READY TO COMMIT TO CHANGE

Now it is time to review your attitudes, beliefs and activity and fitness levels. Have you become committed to an increase in your physical activity? Go back to your list of advantages and disadvantages of becoming more active. Are there items you want to revise? Do you want to add or delete anything? What are your reasons for remaining sedentary? Think through the issues and make a conscious decision. Do not allow failure to make a decision to determine something this important. If you do not arrive at a carefully considered and thoughtful decision about your physical activity and continue with your current habits, your lack of a decision is actually a decision to stay sedentary. Hopefully, your deliberations will convince you to go the next step. Give the next chapter a try. It should not be difficult to make some of the lifestyle changes recommended there.

Good Luck!!!

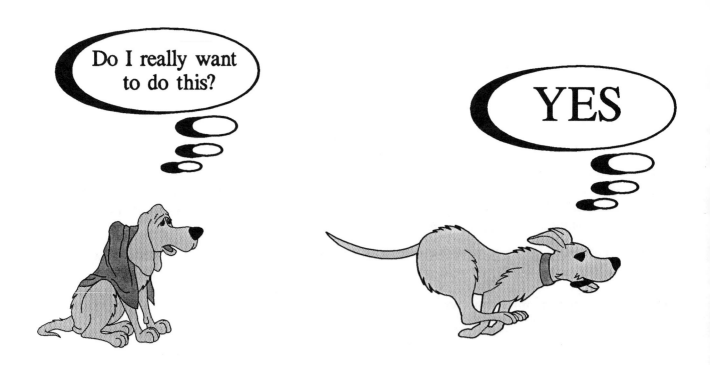

Chapter 3

GETTING STARTED

I hope that by now you are ready to become a more active person. The approach taken here is different from that of most other books on exercise. Current exercise books range from a recent best seller that claimed there were no health benefits of exercise, to books that focus on very detailed and high levels of exercise prescription. It is clear that scientific research confirms the important health benefits resulting from regular physical activity. One of the most important recent findings, from our research and from others, is that moderate levels of exercise and fitness offer considerable advantages for improved health. There are 30 to 50 million adult Americans who could significantly improve their health if they were more active and fit. If you are one of them, this chapter will help get you started. The emphasis is on simple ways to build more activity into your daily life.

THE PROCESS OF BEHAVIOR CHANGE

Changing habits is not easy, at least for most people. Although no single technique works for everyone, you can find ways to change your habits to include more physical activity. A few general guidelines may be helpful to you as you begin to change your behavior. For most people, habit change is not unplanned and spontaneous. It is generally a gradual process and usually takes practice and repeated attempts.

Some people can make behavior changes quickly. We call this type of change the "cold turkey" technique. The person makes a conscious decision to change and consistently adheres to the decision until the old behavioral pattern is eliminated or replaced by a new pattern. "Cold turkey" probably works better for a habit you are trying to stop, such as smoking, than one you are trying to add, such as exercise.

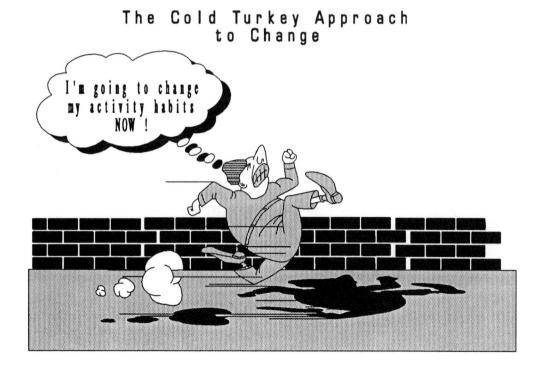

Case Example

Dan Stops Smoking

I was attending a scientific meeting several years ago and went to a lecture by one of the leading researchers on the topic of smoking and health. The lecturer was one of the scientists in the 1950s who first showed increased cardiovascular disease, cancer, and all-cause death rates in smokers. During the question-and-answer session, someone asked him if he had ever been a smoker. "Yes," he replied, "almost 85% of my generation of American men smoked regularly at some time in their lives." The questioner then asked why he had quit. "I stopped on the day we analyzed the first set of death certificates. When I observed the much higher death rates in smokers," he said, "I threw away my pack of cigarettes, and I haven't smoked since."

Some people can make "cold turkey" health behavior changes as Dan did with smoking. If you can do it, great. Unfortunately, this method does not work well for many people. Consider how well you know yourself. Can you make abrupt changes, or do you need to gradually build a new set of behaviors? You need to give this some thought and perhaps some trials, to find out what works best for you.

Developing Your Plan For Change

The process I recommend involves thinking about change and your reasons for it, obtaining information, increasing your motivation to change, and making a specific plan based on your own personal strengths and sources of support. At this point, you need to develop a plan for how you will attempt the change. Please complete the form on the following page. Once your plan is complete, you will be ready to implement the plan. There may be times when the plan does not provide the exact results you want the first time, so you may need to make adjustments to "fine tune" the plan after you evaluate of your progress. You may find that you need to revise your plan. If you find your plan worked well for you, more ambitious goals many need to be developed. When you reach this point, try a new (revised or extended) plan. Learn from your setbacks and build on your successes. Eventually, you will incorporate the changes into your life, and you will be off to a healthier and happier lifestyle.

Start Slowly, But Maybe Not This Slowly.

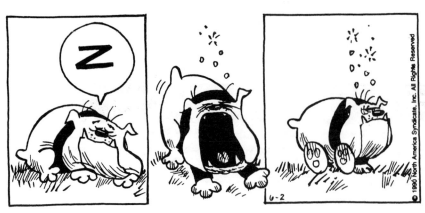
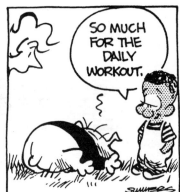

My Plan for Change

1. _____

2. _____

3. _____

4. _____

5. _____

6. _____

7. _____

8. _____

9. _____

Begin with Small Changes

Most people find it difficult to make major changes in behavior all at once. A better strategy is to make a small change, incorporate it into your lifestyle, and then make another change. Over time, you can reshape your behavior. It doesn't matter if it takes weeks or months to achieve an acceptable physical activity level. Many people have been sedentary for decades, so taking a year to restructure physical activity habits is fine. I hope that by now, you can see the many positive benefits of a more active lifestyle. To achieve these benefits, physical activity needs to be added to your permanent lifestyle.

A common problem with sudden changes in behavior, is that they are hard to maintain, and people tend to go off their "program." Try not to think of the recommendations here as a "program." Instead, begin to convert to a more active lifestyle and to view yourself as an exerciser. This doesn't mean that you are necessarily going to become a marathon runner, but that you are no longer going to be sedentary.

CASE EXAMPLE

Brad and the Woodpile

Fireplaces and wood-burning stoves are popular again. However, some of us do not find them so romantic. I grew up in a poor family on a farm in Kansas. In those days, if you were well off, you heated your home with fuel oil. We used wood-burning stoves. This meant finding dead trees along the creek bottom in the late summer and early fall and sawing them into stove-size pieces.

Everyone works in a farm family. My middle brother and I helped Dad milk the cows and feed the livestock. My youngest brother, Brad, was responsible for keeping the woodbox on the back porch filled. One fall, when Brad was about seven years old, an uncle came one Saturday to help us saw wood for the coming winter. As you may imagine, it takes an enormous pile of wood to heat a draughty old farmhouse through a Kansas winter.

When we finished sawing wood that evening, the pile of wood was as big as a house. Brad came up with his wagon to take the night's wood supply down to the house. My uncle said to him, "How long do you think it will take you to get that entire woodpile on the back porch?" You have never seen such a crestfallen boy. He had never considered that eventually he would haul the whole woodpile to the house.

What does this have to do with physical activity? Well, it illustrates the principle of breaking behavior into small units. Eventually my brother hauled all the wood to the house. And eventually you can accumulate enough physical activity to have an impact.

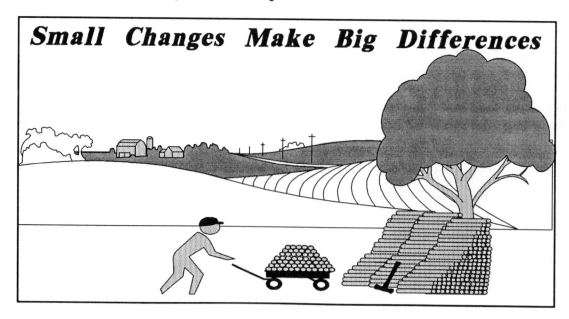

Small Changes Make Big Differences

SEEK OPPORTUNITIES TO SPEND ENERGY

The first step towards a more active life should be relatively painless. Just think of your body as a machine; your task is to use it. You want to use up more fuel by spending energy in small chunks. How do you do that?

One way is to take the stairs instead of the elevator or escalator, especially if you are only going two or three floors. Climbing stairs rates as a very hard activity on our physical activity assessment scale. This means that you burn 10 times more calories climbing stairs than you do resting. Riding an elevator, however, is only slightly more vigorous than resting. Also, taking the stairs is usually faster than waiting for an elevator. Are you really so tired that you can't spend 30 seconds walking up a couple of flights? Condition yourself to think, "I do not take elevators unless I am going more than three floors or if I can't find the stairs."

When you have the time, consider climbing the stairs even if you are going more than three floors. Some people plan to climb 10, 20, or more floors from the parking garage to their office as a part of their efforts to increase energy expenditure. If you work on the 60th floor, you might take the elevator to the 50th or 55th floor and take the stairs the rest of the way. How many flights of stairs can you routinely build into your day? If you can accumulate 10 or 15 minutes of stair climbing a day, it can have an important impact on your physical activity score.

Look for opportunities at work to spend more calories. Walk across the hall to speak to a colleague rather than call on the telephone. Stand up and move around your office while reading a letter or memo. If you supervise other employees, "supervision by walking around" may be a good supervisory practice, and it also burns some calories. Besides this, you will likely find that these very short exercise opportunities make you feel refreshed. I am not suggesting that you spend all day walking around; your boss may not like that. But you may be surprised at how often you can incorporate some movement, or at least some standing, into your routine.

Don't be too eager to use labor-saving devices at home for house and yard work. When we bought our last lawn mower, we purchased the old-fashioned, reel push-type. It really doesn't take any longer, and it provides an exercise opportunity once a week in the summer. It also has some other advantages: it isn't noisy, you can start early and not wake your neighbors, you don't have to buy gas, and its cheaper. Another activity you can build into your life is raking the leaves in the fall. Don't pay your teenage neighbor or a lawn service - you need the exercise more than they do.

Consider, too, whether you can reorganize your housework to spend more energy. That may not make it any more enjoyable, but at least you get some of your exercise while doing a necessary task.

You may think that these suggestions will not make much difference in your overall activity level. But you may be surprised. Don't overlook the cumulative aspect of building in some these opportunities. Remember Brad and the woodpile. A few calories here, a few there, do add up. Keep in mind that sitting burns more calories than lying, standing burns more than sitting,

Spend more energy doing your chores

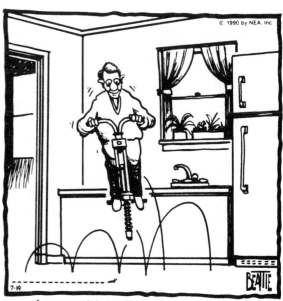

A pogo stick turns roach extermination into beneficial aerobic exercise.

55

moving about burns more than standing, and so on. Another reason for taking this approach is to restructure your concept of yourself as an exerciser. Think of yourself as active, and look for chances to prove it.

Many of the above suggestions can be accomplished within the context of other activities. And when you incorporate exercise into your daily routine, you are achieving two things at once. You are getting needed exercise and accomplishing needed tasks. This incorporation approach to increasing your activity is efficient. You do not have to go to an exercise facility, change clothes, or shower. The ideas presented here are only suggestions; they may or may not fit into your daily routine. As you analyze your own routine, I am confident you can find similar opportunities. Take a moment to think about it, and jot down a few ways in which you can increase the amount of energy you expend, and caloried you burn, by becoming more active. In the box below, list at least five things you can do over the next week to increase your energy output. Be sure not to include those activities you are already doing. Remember, we are looking for new opportunities to spend energy.

Increasing My Energy Output

1. _____

2. _____

3. _____

4. _____

5. _____

The Two-Minute Walk

Take a Walk!

The opportunities to increase energy expenditure discussed above can give you a good start to becoming more active. But you should also try to build in some specific exercise sessions. Start with planning for a two-minute walk. This can be done almost anytime and anywhere. Just set aside two minutes for brisk walking. Get off your bus one block early and walk to your office. Walk a block or two down the street for lunch rather than going across the street. Go out for a two-minute walk before breakfast. Walk down the hall on your coffee break. Take a two-minute walk during a TV commercial. Some of these breaks from work or from sitting will be refreshing and will make you feel better immediately. If you can build several in during the day, the cumulative effect can begin to make a difference in your activity score and in your physical fitness.

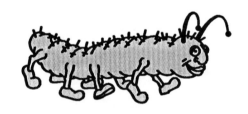

Think about how you can build a two-minute walk into your day. List in the chart on the next page, when you plan to take the two-minute break and how many times a day you will do this exercise initially. My suggestion is that you plan on three to five, two-minute walks a day, but you should make up your own mind. Be realistic. It is more important at this stage to develop a feasible plan and to be successful than it is to get a lot of exercise.

My Plans for a Two-Minute Walks

1. _____

2. _____

3. _____

4. _____

5. _____

I plan to initially build in _____ two-minute walks each day.

DECREASE SEDENTARY ACTIVITIES

There is nothing inherently bad with watching TV, reading, or playing cards. These kinds of activities are relaxing and are important recreational outlets. The problem arises when individuals spend an excessive amount of time in these types of sedentary activities. TV viewing hardly burns more calories than sleeping, and when you do it for several hours a day, which is typical for most Americans, you are losing opportunities to be active. It's a bit like children drinking soft drinks with meals. Soft drinks are not necessarily bad for children, but if they are substituted for milk, the children may be missing some essential nutrients.

One obvious way to become more physically active is to reduce the time spent in very sedentary activities. Take a moment to estimate how many hours of your leisure time are spent sitting. Using the chart on the next page, make a list of these activities and how much time you typically spend on them each day. After you complete the list, develop a plan to reduce the number of hours for at least one activity. Specify what you will substitute in place of the activity you will reduce.

Decrease Sedentary Activities

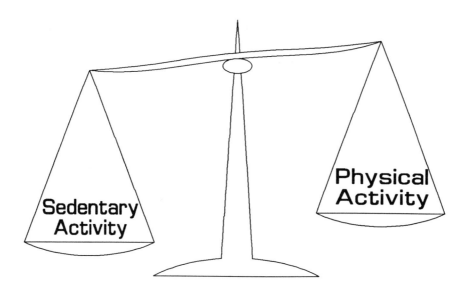

My Very Sedentary Leisure Time Activities

Activity	Hours/Day
1. _____	_____
2. _____	_____
3. _____	_____
4. _____	_____
5. _____	_____

I plan to reduce activity #1 by _____ hours/day next week.

   I will substitute _____.

I plan to reduce activity #2 by _____ hours/day next week.

   I will substitute _____.

I plan to reduce activity #3 by _____ hours/day next week.

   I will substitute _____.

I plan to reduce activity #4 by _____ hours/day next week.

   I will substitute _____.

I plan to reduce activity #5 by _____ hours/day next week.

   I will substitute _____.

Try this substitution for the next week, then evaluate your success, and either revise or extend your plan for the following week. Do not attempt to make drastic reductions in activities you enjoy. It is important to be successful in your plan, so make it realistic.

OVERCOMING BARRIERS

There are innumerable reasons for not making a behavior change. There is never a good time for it. You are too busy at work. The holidays are coming up. Your daughter is getting married. You are going on vacation. Your mother is coming for a visit. You can probably think of many more reasons. Since there may never be a good time to start, one time is as good as the next. You might as well start now to make changes in your physical activity habits. Following are some suggestions on how to overcome barriers to change. I'm sure that you can think of additional techniques to getting past these hurdles.

Lack of Time

"I just don't have time to exercise." This is probably the most frequently stated excuse for not being more active. Let's examine this issue in more detail and see if there are ways you can find the time.

A few years ago, a survey on exercise habits and related issues was done with a representative sample of American men and women. Participants were asked about what types and amounts of exercise they regularly participated in. Some people did absolutely nothing and were labeled sedentary. Another group, admittedly much smaller, regularly participated in about five hours of vigorous exercise each week. These individuals were the joggers, enthusiastic tennis players, bicyclists, and others engaged in vigorous sports. The survey participants were also asked several other questions about their lifestyle. One question asked how much leisure time they had each week. Both the sedentary and vigorously active groups reported nearly identical amounts of leisure time, about 24 hours a week.

What is the lesson we can learn from this survey? We all have the same number of hours at our disposal each week, 168. But we do have the same choice of how we spend them. Certain tasks are prerequisite, such as sleeping, working, domestic duties, and so on, but we all have some discretionary time. The individuals in the survey described above had more than 20 hours a week, on the average. Different people make different decisions about how to use that time. Some individuals with very demanding jobs still manage to find time for physical activity. Several of our recent U.S. Presidents had regular exercise programs. President Carter was a jogger, President Ford swam and played sports, President Reagan did calisthenics and other activities, and President Bush jogs and generally leads a very active life. What job is more demanding and time-consuming than that of President of the United States? Other examples of active individuals abound. Business executives, housewives, scientists, and other professionals jog, play vigorous sports, or are otherwise quite active. If these individuals can find time in their schedules for exercise, so can the rest of us.

Building in time for yourself to exercise is largely a matter of assigning priorities. You do have some leisure time. You spend some time reading, watching TV, daydreaming, etc. Which of these activities can you cut back so you can get in your four, two-minute walks each day?

The type and amount of exercise recommended here are not terribly time-consuming. Simply take the time to fit some new activities into your daily routine, and take a few two-minute walks. Work on giving exercise a high enough priority so that you fit it in.
Make the time!

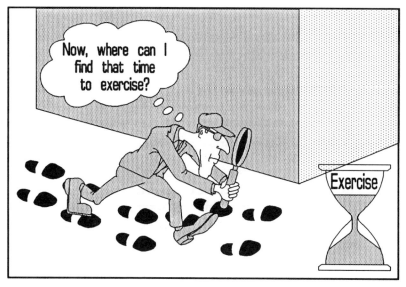

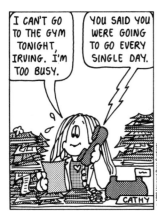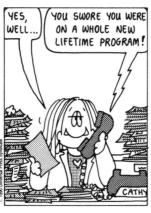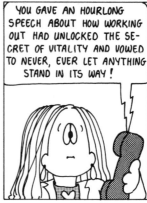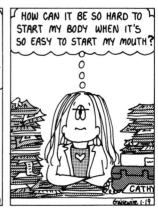

Lack of Skill

Some people are sedentary because they have never developed physical activity skills. They may lack some of the physical attributes necessary for athletic success, or they may have never had the interest to develop sports skills. These individuals may lack self-confidence and may be afraid that others will laugh at them if they try to play a particular sport. Many fit the example of George.

CASE EXAMPLE

George the Klutz

A friend of mine, George, was taught to hate physical activity. He is not very well coordinated, and wasn't good at sports. Consequently, other children laughed at him. He was always chosen last in games, and when he did play he made mistakes and played poorly. His physical education teachers didn't help. Mistakes in PE class produced orders to do push-ups and run laps. Thus, over his formative years, George was conditioned to think of himself as a klutz and to dislike any type of exercise or sports.

As an adult, George was able to realize that some regular physical activity is a good health habit. He resolved to become more active, even though he still hated exercise. He convinced himself that he would start walking with his friend Mary, who lived in the next apartment. Mary went out every weekday morning for a 15-minute walk before breakfast. George made the commitment to join her. He decided to view it as 15 minutes of preventive medicine that he would take for his health. At first, he found it hard to comply. He still hated exercise, and he didn't especially like getting up a little earlier, but he persisted. Mary expected George to walk with her, and he wasn't the type of a person to let a friend down.

George and Mary are in the same profession and have many of the same cultural interests. They disagree violently on politics. They have plenty to talk about on their walks, and the conversations are usually stimulating. George has yet to convince Mary that supply-side economics works, and she can't get him to see the logic of gun control, but they are still friends. George's morning walk meets both his need for physical activity and his need for socialization. The enjoyment of Mary's company and conversation is the "spoonful of sugar" that makes "the exercise pill go down."

Mary took an extended business trip a few months ago. George knew that he would miss her company, but he was surprised to discover that he also missed the brisk walk. He slept in the first morning Mary was gone. While getting ready to go to work, he realized how good he had felt after his walks with Mary. During the remainder of Mary's trip, George found himself walking alone every morning. To this day, George is still not very good at sports, but he is now an excellent exerciser.

Do you have a long-standing dislike of exercise? Can you follow George's example and make a change? Think of ways you can make exercise more enjoyable to overcome unpleasant memories or associations. List in the chart below five things you can do to make exercise more enjoyable for you.

Making Exercise More Enjoyable

1. _____

2. _____

3. _____

4. _____

5. _____

CASE EXAMPLE

Jane and Her Seat Belt

My wife generally has excellent health behaviors. She eats a nutritious diet, runs regularly, doesn't smoke, and now wears seat belts when in the car. This last behavior, however, is a recent adoption. For many years, she only wore seat belts sporadically. Although she knew the data on seat belts and survival rates from auto accidents, she frequently failed to fasten her seat belt.

Why do you suppose she made the behavior change? The reason was an environmental factor. When we met, Jane had a new 1964 VW Beetle. She was quite attached to it and drove it until our son inherited it in his senior year of high school in 1987. The Beetle was a wonderful car for its time, especially for young families with limited funds. But it did have some drawbacks. The heating system was hard to adjust, and the seat belts were hard to fasten.

For those of you who don't have a 1964 Beetle, the seat belt connector on the inside of the seat is on the end of a short section of seat belt; it was not attached to a rigid support. Therefore, whenever you tried to fasten your seat belt, you had to find the inboard end. Unfortunately, the belt was frequently under the seat. When you pushed the seat back forward to let someone into the back seat, the inboard belt usually got tangled in the seat support. If you wanted to buckle up, you sometimes had to get out of the seat, hold the seat forward, untangle the belt, get back in, and hope that it had not fallen under the front seat again. Jane did not wear her seat belt most times because it was inconvenient. But her new car has a much more user friendly seat belt system, and now she is always belted in.

Think about whether environmental factors affect your behavior. Are you sedentary because it is inconvenient to be more active? Can you think of ways to restructure your environment or your schedule to make exercise more convenient and less of a hassle? I emphasize walking because it tends to be more convenient than other exercise. It does not require equipment or a companion, and walking in a controlled environment, such as a shopping mall, eliminates climatic problems and safety hazards.

Making Exercise More Convenient

The environment in many of our urban areas is not conducive to physical activity. In some areas there are no sidewalks. You may feel that it is not safe to walk on the streets. Also, many people find that it is much easier to drive on an errand than it is to walk. Our culture is oriented towards the automobile and away from human power.

Have you noticed that in some situations there are more people walking than in others? If you go to New Orleans on vacation and visit the French Quarter, you will probably walk more than when you are at home. It is difficult to drive there, the streets are full of people walking, and there are many sights to see and things to do. Activity levels seem to be higher in some communities because of the extensive network of bicycle paths, barriers on the streets to make direct routes by car impossible, and a general atmosphere of an active populace. Environmental, physical, and cultural factors can be major barriers to changes in health behavior. The lesson here is for you to become aware of these barriers and recognize those factors that are barriers to you. List below some of the barriers that keep you from exercising.

```
+---------------------------------------------------------------+
|        What Barriers Are Keeping You From Exercising?         |
|  1. _____  |
|                                                               |
|  2. _____  |
|                                                               |
|  3. _____  |
|                                                               |
|  4. _____  |
|                                                               |
|  5. _____  |
|                                                               |
+---------------------------------------------------------------+
```

List below five ways in which you can alter your environment or schedule to make physical activity more convenient. Identify at least one that you will implement next week.

```
+---------------------------------------------------------------+
|           Ways to Make Exercise More Convenient               |
|  1. _____  |
|                                                               |
|  2. _____  |
|                                                               |
|  3. _____  |
|                                                               |
|  4. _____  |
|                                                               |
|  5. _____  |
|                                                               |
|  I will implement # _____ next week.                      |
+---------------------------------------------------------------+
```

In this chapter, I've given you several suggestions on how to get started with making changes in your physical activity. Most of the suggestions are very simple and are designed to be built into your daily activities. The two-minute walks can help you get started with a specific exercise plan. Important principles underlying the suggestions include starting slowly and building change in small increments and your involvement in the planning and implementation of your more active lifestyle. Please feel free to substitute some of your own ideas. You are the one who must make the approach work for you.

You should now have some basic ideas about the strategies you plan to use to increase your physical activity. Several general approaches have been reviewed briefly so far: *cold turkey*, *environmental planning*, *time management*, *social support*, and *behavioral manipulations*. Which of these do you plan to use? Make a list below.

My strategies for increasing physical activity are:

_____

_____

_____

_____

Good luck in trying to make changes. Do not continue on to the next chapter until you have tried out the exercise plan you developed for initial implementation. You need to have some trials, build on your successes, and modify plans that did not work. Some people may be able to achieve this in several days; for others, this may take as long as a few weeks. Keep at it. You're on your way.

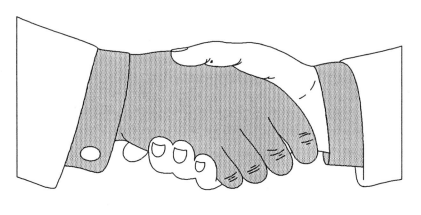

Good Luck!

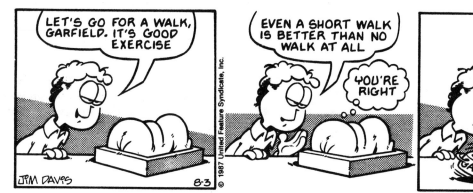
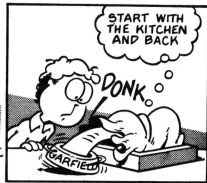

Chapter 4

MAKING PROGRESS

I hope that you have been successful in carrying out the first phase of your plan to become more physically active. In the previous chapter there were several suggestions for gradually changing from a sedentary to an active lifestyle. What progress have you made? One suggestion was to seek ways at home and at work to increase your energy expenditure. Have you been using the stairs rather than the elevator? Do you now park farther away from the door at your office? What changes have you implemented? Please note below the changes you have attempted and whether you were successful.

Evaluation of My Activity Plan

Ways of Increasing Energy Output Both in Daily Life & During a Planned Exercise Time

1. _____
2. _____
3. _____
4. _____
5. _____

Evaluation: Degree of Success

1. _____
2. _____
3. _____
4. _____
5. _____

If some of your attempts did not meet with success, do not be discouraged. Try something else. Continue the techniques that were successful, and try to increase the frequency of these activities. Make a new list of ways you will try to increase your energy output in the coming weeks.

Ways I Will Increase My Energy Output

1. _____
2. _____
3. _____
4. _____
5. _____

Now might be a good time to consider rewarding yourself for increasing your level of activity and your energy output. Set a level or number of episodes of increases in expenditure that you will try to meet each week. If you meet your goal, reward yourself. The reward need not be expensive or elaborate. Treat yourself to a movie, buy a new shirt that you have wanted but felt that you did not deserve, or enjoy a favorite television show. Try to avoid rewards that are food oriented. This is especially important if you are on a weight management program. Set a specific goal, have a specific reward in mind, and if you meet the goal, take satisfaction from the reward. Use your imagination. You should know what type of reward will work for you. List below your goal and your reward.

MY GOAL

**My Goal for Increasing
My Energy Expenditure Is:**

_____

_____

_____

**If I Meet My Goal,
I Will Reward Myself With:**

_____

_____

_____

MY REWARD

THE TWO-MINUTE WALK

The Two-Minute Walk

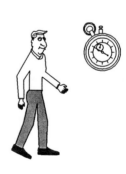

In the last chapter, you set a goal for taking a certain number of two-minute walks each day. How have you done? Were you able to meet your target? Review your successes and your setbacks. I hope that you found it easy to take the short walks and to build them into your schedule. But if you did not, try to analyze why your plans did not work and develop a new approach.

Do not be discouraged if you were not 100% successful. Remember, behavior change takes time. You do not need to make major changes all at the same time. The important thing is to have some success in changing your behavior, and build on those changes. Remember Brad and the woodpile; he took a little wood each day. Eventually the whole pile was moved to the back porch. You can do the same in adopting the two-minute walks.

Consider how many two-minute walks you have been able to include in your day. How many did you do last week? Plan to increase the number next week. If the opportunities for walks you selected initially are working, continue and try to extend some of the walks to three minutes. Seek other times to add more short walks to your day in the coming weeks. Below, list the plans that were successful and can be extended, and add new opportunities for the future.

My Revised Plans for Two (or Three) Minute Walks

1. _____

2. _____

3. _____

4. _____

5. _____

Next week I will build in _____ two- or three-minute walks each day.

Strive to implement these revised plans for short walks next week. Build on your successes with small increments. You are on your way to a more physically active and fit way of life!

SEARCHING FOR REINFORCERS

Anyone who has ever trained a puppy knows behavior that receives reinforcement is likely to be repeated. We're not saying you're a puppy, but the puppy example does apply. The rewards discussed above are one kind of reinforcement that may help you establish new exercise habits. Reinforcers do not have to be tangible rewards. A supportive comment from someone else can reinforce your desire to maintain your exercise, just as "good dog," coupled with a pat, encourages the puppy to sit or stay.

Your own thoughts and self-talk can also reinforce your behavior. Doesn't increasing your physical activity make you feel better? Even the two-minute walk can relieve tension, relax you, and clear your mind. Focus on how good it makes you feel.

Join the crowd.
The two-minute walks do make you feel great!

Think of your new image. Can you begin to see yourself as more fit and able to do more things? Enjoy this new perception of yourself as a high functioning individual.

Review some of the other immediate benefits of activity. Think of the calories you are burning. Imagine the beneficial effects on your muscle cells. They are becoming more sensitive to insulin, better adapted to performing muscular work, and perhaps are becoming stronger. What other benefits have you experienced?

One group of middle school teachers I know searches for coins on the ground as they take their walk after school. Another friend, who has run several dozen marathons, has a large jar into which he puts the coins he finds on his runs. His collection is truly impressive and includes coins from many countries.

Another approach is to become more observant, and enjoy the environment. Take pleasure in the flower gardens and admire beautiful or unusual homes. My wife used to run with an architect who was always looking for different examples of how space was used.

Consider the long-term benefits of more activity as well. Remember that the more you improve your fitness, at least up to a point, the more you are lowering your risk for serious chronic disease or death. Also, think of how much you are increasing your ability to function. You will be able to do more without becoming fatigued. You will be better able to handle routine daily tasks. And, if you get the opportunity to go to Bermuda or Hawaii, you will be fit enough to enjoy snorkeling, take a walk along the beach, or do the limbo.

HAVING TROUBLE GETTING STARTED

Are you having trouble taking the first step to becoming more physically active? Good intentions are often not enough - you must begin to move. On the following pages, I offer some suggestions that may be helpful:

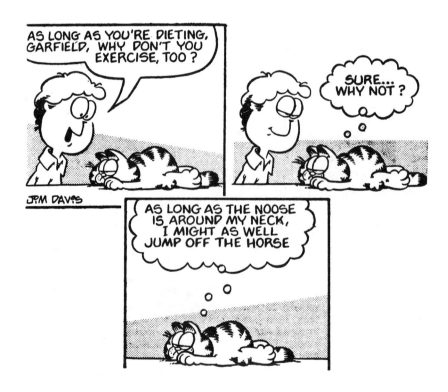

Twenty-Five Ways To Get Moving

1. Take the baby for a stroll.

2. Put your exercise clothes on when you get up, and don't take them off until you get some exercise.

3. Make a date to do something active with a friend.

4. Ask a friend or family member to give you a call to remind you to exercise.

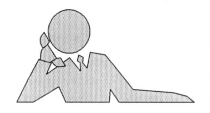

5. Set your alarm to remind you to take a two-minute walk.

6. Refuse to eat lunch until after you take at least a two-minute walk.

7. Plan some errands that require walking for your lunch hour.

8. Take your dog for a walk; he or she also needs the exercise. If you train your dog, your dog will remind you to walk.

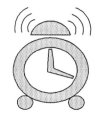

9. If you don't have a dog, borrow a neighbor's.

10. Find a partner for a game of Frisbee.

11. Take up an active hobby.

12. Enroll in a folk dance class.

13. Mow your lawn twice a week.

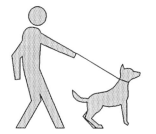

14. Sweep your sidewalk and patio.

15. Put some 1950s music on the stereo, and dance to some rock and roll. You don't need a partner; dance by yourself if necessary.

16. Walk a few blocks to visit a shut in.

17. Volunteer to take the scouts camping.

18. Help lead a nursery field trip to the zoo.

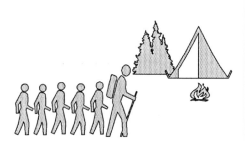

19. Walk and talk with your child or spouse. There are no phones or television to interrupt your conversation.

20. Play hopscotch with neighborhood children.

21. Plan short bicycle rides.

22. Go for a walk during TV commercials.

23. Limit your television watching by 10% and substitue this time with some physical activity.

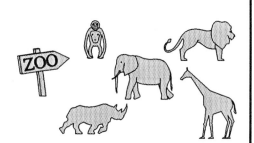

24. Take a two-minute walk before going to bed.

25. Join a walking club.

Now that you have seen my list of activities, it is now time to come up with your own. On the chart below, make a list of twenty-five things that you can do to get you moving. Listing the activities does not mean you will do them all at the same time. As you continue in your activity program, refer back to this list. You will be amazed how helpful it will become.

My Twenty-Five Ways to Get Moving

_____

Graphing Your Activities

Research shows that keeping records of your behavior helps you make and maintain changes. The act of record-keeping reinforces the behavior change, and the permanent record can be used for planning and guidance in your program. Record-keeping can be simple or elaborate. What you do should depend on your personality, your desires, and what seems to work for you.

There are some simple approaches to record-keeping that you can use. The specific technique depends partly on what changes you are trying to make. For example, if you are trying to increase stair climbing instead of using the elevator, simply record how many flights you climb each day. You can carry a 3 X 5 card in your pocket and make a tally mark each time you take the stairs. At the end of the day, or end of the week, transfer the tally to a notebook where you can record or plot weekly totals. You may want to construct a simple graph. Watching the line march up the graph as you increase a behavior can be reinforcing.

A more elaborate example of record-keeping is to graph your daily energy expenditure. Use the procedure explained in Chapter 2 for calculating your energy expenditure in calories per kilogram of body weight per day. Remember, if you are sedentary, your expenditure score will be in the low 30s. Your goal should be to score into the high 30s on this measure. Gradually increase your daily caloric expenditure to 38 to 40 calories per kilogram.

Nancy used to be a very sedentary individual. She adopted some of the ideas in this book to help her increase her daily activity level. Nancy is the type of person who enjoyed getting more involved in her activity progress and immediately began to calculate her energy expenditure. She relished plotting her progress and seeing continuous improvement in her scores. Nancy was successful in increasing her activity level and gained more and more self-esteem as she watched her progress. An example of Nancy's energy expenditure graph is shown below.

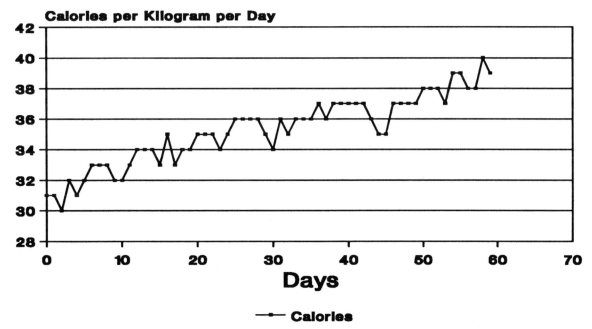

Change in Caloric Expenditure

Note that Nancy's progress was not consistently upward. This is to be expected. You will not proceed without interruptions towards your goal. The overall progress shown in Nancy's graph is one of steady improvement. You may have more or less difficulty than this person. You may make progress for a few weeks, then actually go all the way back down to your starting point. This is not a disaster; you simply need to get back on track. The goal should be, that in a year from now, you are consistently expending more energy over a week's time than you are now.

IS YOUR FITNESS IMPROVING

Are you getting more physically fit? If you have been successful in increasing your activity over a period of several weeks, your body may be adapting physiologically. You may have noticed that it is easier to climb a couple of flights of stairs without becoming short of breath. You may not be as tired at the end of the day. Doing your weekend chores in the house and yard may not be as fatiguing as it was before. If you are noticing some of these changes, then your fitness is improving.

If you want to more formally test yourself and quantify your progress, you may want to repeat one of the fitness tests described in Chapter 2. If you did not take a test initially, of course, you cannot take one now to note progress, but it might still be worthwhile to take a test at this time in order to monitor your progress in the future. If you don't want to bother with testing, that is fine. We all have different ways of doing things.

You may repeat one of the fitness tests and note no progress. Don't be concerned. You may not have been exercising long enough, or perhaps you haven't yet made sufficient changes in your physical activity to produce a fitness response. These simple field tests are not as sensitive as a laboratory test in measuring fitness, so it is possible that the self-administered test cannot detect small changes in your fitness. Just remember, the most important thing is to gradually made changes in your physical activity habits. It doesn't matter how quickly you progress, just keep it up. It is more important to gradually make permanent changes than to make a major change that you are unable to sustain.

REVIEW

It may be useful to review your attitudes, beliefs, and reasons for wanting to become more physically active. I suggest that you go back to Chapter 1, and scan the advantages and disadvantages of exercise you listed at that time. Spend a few minutes going over the pros and cons of becoming more active. Have your ideas or beliefs changed? Does this have any potential impact on your attempts to become more active and fit? Can you explain to a friend how and why exercise is beneficial? Why do you want to become more active? Do you want to live longer? Do you want to be able to do more and have more fun? Do you want to avoid being left out, as Patty was?

You are in charge of your health. You must make the decisions to alter your activity, and you must be responsible for developing and implementing your plan. I can give some suggestions, but you are in charge. ***You can do it!*** Millions of people have successfully made changes in health behaviors, and have reaped the benefits. You can too.

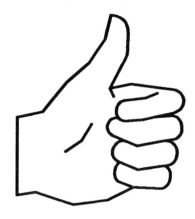

Chapter 5

NUTRITION AND EXERCISE

Chronic diseases, such as cardiovascular disease and cancer, are the major health problems of our society. These and other leading causes of death and disability have multiple factors leading to their development. Poor health habits are the primary contributors to the risks of chronic disease. The focus of this book, exercise and physical fitness, is one of the most important lifestyle factors to consider in connection with these diseases. But exercise is not the only important factor. The high-calorie, high-fat, and high-sodium diet consumed by many also contributes to numerous health problems. If you are also interested in improving your nutritional habits, this chapter will provide some basic information. A more detailed presentation of this topic is available in *The LEARN Program for Weight Control* by Kelly D. Brownell, Ph.D.

DOES GOOD EXERCISE
OVERCOME BAD NUTRITION

I have often been asked, "If I exercise vigorously and frequently, do I still have to be concerned about my diet?" The answer is yes. Regular exercise and a high level of physical fitness help to reduce your risk of premature death, but a healthy diet is still important. Let me illustrate with some data from our Aerobics Center Longitudinal Study, which I discussed briefly in Chapter 1.

In this study, more than 13,000 men and women were followed for a little longer than eight years after their examinations at the Institute in Dallas. All of these individuals had an exercise test on a treadmill as part of their examination. These treadmill test results were used to group the study participants into low, moderate, and high fitness groups. We found that all-cause, cardiovascular disease, and cancer death rates decline sharply from the low to high fitness groups. The all-cause death rates (deaths per 10,000) for the fitness groups are 64, 27, 20 in men and 40, 16, 7 in women.

We do not have comprehensive data about the diets of the subjects in our study, but we did measure blood cholesterol. High levels of blood cholesterol are primarily due to a diet high in fat and cholesterol. Blood cholesterol levels are a good indicator for certain dietary patterns. It was no surprise, in our study, to discover that persons with high levels of blood cholesterol were more likely to die during the follow-up period. This relationship has been demonstrated before in many other studies.

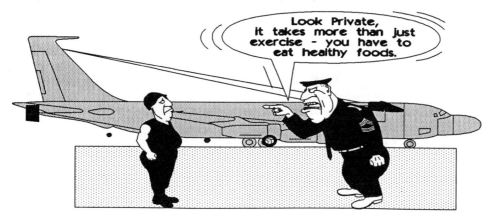

We also were interested in evaluating the independent contributions of fitness and cholesterol on risk of early death. To do this, all-cause death rates across fitness categories were examined in men and women with high levels of blood cholesterol. Patients with a blood cholesterol of greater than 260 milligrams per deciliter of blood were classified at high risk on cholesterol. This level of blood cholesterol falls into the high risk category as specified by such groups as the National Institutes of Health, the American Heart Association, and the National Cholesterol Education Program. All-cause death rates for men with high cholesterol were calculated for the three fitness groups. We did not have enough women with high cholesterol to do a similar analysis, so only data on men are presented. The results for men are shown in the figure below.

Men with Cholesterol > 260 mg/dl

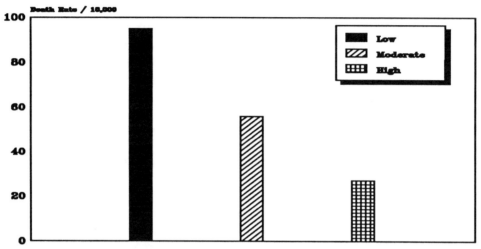

Physical Fitness Groups

Higher levels of physical fitness appear to be protective in these men with high levels of blood cholesterol. The death rate for the fit men with high cholesterol was 27 per 10,000 and this was less than one-third the rate (95 per 10,000) of the low fit men.

But more to the point of this section, the high fit men with high cholesterol (death rate of 27 per 10,000) were at higher risk than high fit men with low cholesterol (below 200 mg/dl). The death rate for these fit men with low cholesterol is not shown on the figure, but it was only 14 per 10,000. Thus, high fit men were less likely to die; but there was still a strong gradient within this group across cholesterol levels. The fit men with high cholesterol were about twice as likely to die as the fit men with low cholesterol (death rates of 27 and 14 respectively).

The main point of all these numbers is that both fitness and cholesterol are important predictors of early death. You cannot rely solely on your exercise habits or fitness level to provide optimum benefit. Diet and activity both need your attention.

Another interesting finding from our fitness and cholesterol analyses was that the high fit, high cholesterol men were less likely to die than low fit men with a cholesterol below 200 mg/dl. These low fit, low cholesterol men had a death rate of 68 per 10,000, or more than twice that of the high fit, high cholesterol men (27 per 10,000). This result suggests that high fitness is more protective than low cholesterol; but that is a story for another time, and more research needs to be done in this area.

In summary, exercise and a high level of physical fitness are important for your health, but they cannot eliminate the harmful effects of a poor diet.

Does Diet Change Naturally with Exercise?

Everyone can think of a friend who is fanatical about health habits. The health nut gets a lot of exercise, is a vegetarian, is skinny, does not smoke or use tobacco in any form, always buckles up when in a car, flosses after each meal, and practices meditation three times a day. Observation of such individuals leads us to believe that health habits cluster in individuals, that some follow unhealthy lifestyles and others are extremely health conscious. We have published several studies on whether health behaviors cluster, and the truth is that they do not. Oh, there are a few low correlations between some habits, but the overall relationship is weak. It is surprising, but even the relationship between exercise and smoking is not nearly as strong as you might think.

In our study, we compared the diets of men and women runners to diets of randomly selected community residents who were not exercisers. The 34 men and 27 women runners were running about 35 to 40 miles per week on the average, so they were reasonably dedicated to exercise. The 61 runners and 80 nonexercisers all completed carefully collected three-day diet records, in which all food and beverages consumed were recorded. The food records were reviewed by a nutritionist, entered into a computer, and analyzed to determine dietary composition.

The runners were much leaner, had lower levels of total blood cholesterol, and showed higher levels of HDL-cholesterol (the "good" cholesterol). High levels of total cholesterol have been shown to increase the risk of coronary heart disease. Two components of total cholesterol are HDL and LDL cholesterol. Higher levels of HDL cholesterol are associated with a lower risk of heart disease, while higher levels of LDL, "bad" cholesterol," are associated with higher risk of such disease.

The only dietary difference between the groups' was that the runners had a much higher caloric intake. The men runners consumed about 600 calories more each day than the nonrunners, and the women runners ate about 500 calories more daily than their sedentary peers. These higher caloric intakes are not surprising; after all, the energy for all the running had to come from somewhere.

The amount of total fat, saturated fat, unsaturated fat, cholesterol, protein, and carbohydrate in the diets was essentially identical for the runners and nonrunners. The runners had more favorable blood cholesterol patterns, but that must have been due to their lower body weights and the running itself. We have studied this issue several times over the past decade and continue to come to the same conclusion. Exercisers and nonexercisers seem to eat about the same diets. Therefore, if you want the benefits of a healthful diet, you must plan for it specifically. There does not appear to be anything inherent about exercise that will cause you to naturally convert to better eating habits.

Do Exercisers Need Increased Nutrients?

Some people believe that if you exercise, you have an increased need for many nutrients. Stores selling exercise equipment and some exercise magazines heavily promote food supplements. You may reason that exercise is "burning up" a lot of nutrients, therefore you need to take some vitamin pills or eat special foods. This is unnecessary. A well-balanced diet will supply the essential nutrients your body needs. The only increased dietary need exercisers have is for more calories. Remember the runners' diet study described above. Runners consumed 500-600 more calories a day than nonrunners. The human body is like an automobile. The more miles you cover and the more fuel you burn, the more you have to put into the tank.

Athletes in heavy training need many more calories and may even require supplementation of certain nutrients. It has been suggested that athletes need slightly more protein, iron, and B vitamins in their diet. But this is still controversial and more research is needed. It **is** clear that individuals who are exercising for health and fitness, and are not pushing themselves to the limits of their endurance, do not require special dietary supplementation.

Does Exercise Depress Your Appetite?

There is a widely believed myth that exercise causes you to eat less. As we discussed earlier, more caloric expenditure requires more caloric intake. The Laws of Thermodynamics apply in the human body as they do in the rest of the universe. More exercise creates a demand for more fuel.

There is a second myth that overweight is caused by high caloric intake. This is not true. Per capita caloric intake in the United States has steadily declined during the 20th century, while the population has gotten progressively heavier. How can this be? The answer has to be that there has been an accompanying decline in the number of calories we burn. Think about it. During the early 1900s, the average person led a much more active life. We didn't have as many labor-saving devices in the home, there were many more physically demanding occupations, and there were very few automobiles.

In addition to the population trends described above, current studies also support the notion that overweight is not usually due to overeating. Large surveys show an inverse relationship between caloric intake and body weight. The people who eat the least weigh the most. This observation, and research such as the runners' diet study, led Dr. Peter Wood of Stanford University Medical School to coin the phrase, "Eat more, weigh less." This seemingly paradoxical statement is due to the effect of exercise. In general, someone who eats more calories is physically active. And physical activity has a beneficial impact on weight control.

There is a short-lived effect of a bout of vigorous exercise on appetite. You usually do not want to eat immediately after a five mile run or a few strenuous sets of tennis. Vigorous exercise apparently causes the brain to release a substance that depresses appetite, but *it only lasts for a short time.* This does not effect your overall caloric intake; and as repeatedly stated, more exercise ultimately causes you to eat more. Still, the acute appetite suppressive action of vigorous exercise can be used to your advantage if you are trying to lose weight. When you have a craving for food, take a short bout of vigorous exercise. It may help you deal with the craving.

PRINCIPLES OF GOOD NUTRITION

Residents of the United States have ready access to one of the cheapest, most plentiful, and diverse food supplies ever known on this planet. We spend a smaller percentage of our incomes on food than any other country. Food is everywhere. In any urban or suburban area of the country, you are never more than a very few minutes away from a place where you can obtain something to eat. And the variety is enormous. Our supermarkets have a seemingly endless supply of fresh produce; in most cities, virtually all the world's cuisines are readily available. All this makes it quite easy to obtain a nutritionally adequate diet.

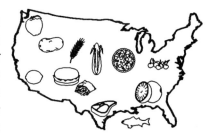

Food is Everywhere !

I may offend the dietitians, but good nutrition is very simple. You do not need a degree in food science to select and consume a well-balanced and healthy diet. Just follow the few simple principles discussed briefly in this section.

The Principal Principle

No, I am not referring to the chief administrator at your neighborhood school. **Principal** means first in rank, and **principle** means a fundamental truth or law, so here I present the most important guideline to a nutritionally adequate diet. And that is balance. Eat a variety of foods. Select widely from the available choices. Dieticians have developed some simple guidelines to help achieve this goal, using the Basic Four Food Groups. The four groups and the minimum number of servings recommended per day are shown on the next page.

The Basic Four Food Groups
(Minimum Daily Requirements)

■ *Fruits and vegetables group--four servings each day.*

Serving Size

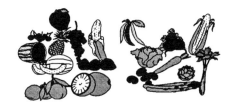
4 Servings Per Day

     1/2 cup cooked or 1 cup raw

     1 orange, small salad

     medium-size potato

■ *Bread and cereal group--four servings each day.*

Serving Size

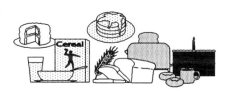
4 Servings Per Day

     1/2 cup cooked cereal, rice, or pasta

     1 slice of bread

     1 ounce of ready-to-eat cereal

■ *Meat group--two servings each day.*

Serving Size

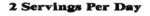
2 Servings Per Day

     1 cup of cooked dry beans or other legumes

     1 cup of nuts or sunflower seeds

     3-4 ounces of meat

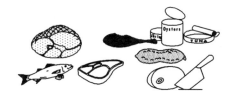

■ *Dairy group--two servings for adults and three to four servings for children or pregnant or lactating women each day.*

Serving Size

2 - 4 Servings Per Day

     1 cup of milk or yogurt

     2 cups of cottage cheese

     1 ounce of cheese

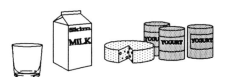

The number of servings you should eat will vary depending on your physical activity. Use the recommendations on the previous page for selecting foods from the four groups. Remember, these are the minimum daily recommended requirements. In addition, the following guidelines from the U. S. Departments of Agriculture and Health and Human Services are recommended:

- **Eat a variety of foods.**

- **Maintain desirable weight.**

- **Avoid too much fat, saturated fat, and cholesterol.**

- **Eat foods with adequate starch and fiber.**

- **Avoid too much sugar.**

- **Avoid too much sodium.**

- **If you drink alcoholic beverages, do so in moderation.**

Many people believe that dieting is like a light switch; they are either "on" or "off." It would be better if we recognized diets and dietary guidelines as a spectrum. Caloric intake can range from 0 to several thousand calories a day. Unless you are in a complete fast, you are not "off" or "on" a diet, but are consuming calories at a particular level. The same reasoning holds for each of the guidelines. Note that many of the guidelines read "avoid too much ..." - they do not stress abstinence of foods. A good strategy is for you to evaluate where you are on a distribution of, let us say, fat intake. Recommended levels of fat intake are about 30% of your total calories from fat. A sizeable proportion of the U. S. population consumes 40% or more of their calories in the form of fat. They would obviously benefit from reducing their fat intake, but they should not eliminate fat from their diet altogether.

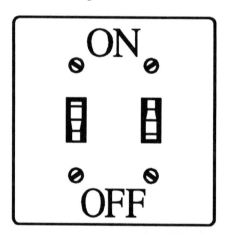

The Diet Switch

Where you should fall on the spectrum of fat intake depends on several factors. The primary one is your level of risk for heart disease. If your cholesterol level is high, perhaps above 240 mg/dl, you may need to restrict your fat intake more than someone with low cholesterol. The presence of other risk factors for coronary heart disease, such as high blood pressure or cigarette smoking, should also be considered. If you have one or more of these other risk factors, it is even more important to reduce your cholesterol level by restricting fat in your diet.

You should evaluate carefully, your personal situation and make decisions about how you plan to implement each of the dietary guidelines. Take into account where you are in meeting a particular recommendation, your overall health status, other specific risk factors, your personal likes and dislikes, and your motivation to make changes.

What Should I Actually Eat?

Recommendations and guidelines are fine, but what you need to do is plan for specific food consumption. People choose foods, not nutrients. Although you can make selection of foods complicated and follow specific formulas in a scientific approach to diet, a few very simple practices can go a long way toward helping you have a more healthful diet.

- **Increase your intake of fresh fruits, vegetables, and whole grains.** It is not that these foods have any magical properties themselves; but if you make these choices, you may reduce the intake of some of the foods that you should avoid. For example, if you eat a grapefruit and cereal for breakfast, you will not be eating sausage, biscuits, and cream gravy.

  Scientists at my institution studied the cholesterol levels of 2,947 men in relation to their typical breakfast pattern. Men who ate cereal for breakfast had cholesterol levels of 210 mg/dl on the average. Men who ate other foods for breakfast had average cholesterols of 217, and men who skipped breakfast had average cholesterols of 222.

  Be careful that you do not negate the beneficial effect of fruits, vegetables, and grains in your diet by the way they are prepared and served. Use low-fat methods of preparation, do not add large amounts of fat, and use skim milk on your cereal.

- **Reduce the amount of fat in your diet.** You should strive to reduce the total number of calories from fat, and pay special attention to reducing saturated fat. Saturated fat is probably the major dietary culprit in terms of impact on blood cholesterol levels. Saturated fat is the fat from animal sources, such as meat and dairy products, and also from certain vegetable oils, such as palm and coconut oil. Except for these oils, saturated fat is solid at room temperature, so any solid fat can be considered saturated.

  The major source of saturated fat for most people is from meat, so perhaps this should be the first place you should attempt changes. A sensible recommendation is to eat no more than about four servings of red meat a week, with each serving limited to about four ounces. With the typical American diet, it is possible to get that quota in a couple of days. Sausage for breakfast, a hamburger for lunch, and a small steak for dinner use three of the four servings in the first day. Another problem with many red meats, including bacon, hamburger, sausage, luncheon meats, and many steaks and roasts, is that they are high in fat. We usually think of steak as a high-protein food, but in many steaks, more than 50% of the total calories are derived from fat.

  Another major source of fat in the typical American diet is dairy products. Most of us love cheese, ice cream, rich sauces made from cream, and other milk- or cream-based foods. Like steak, whole milk is a high-fat, rather than a high-protein food. To make changes, substitute skim milk or low-fat milk and milk products for whole milk and cheeses made with whole milk and cream.

You also have to be alert to hidden fat. Convenience or highly processed foods frequently are high in fat, and much of it is saturated. Fast foods are another prominent source of fat in the diet. A fast food restaurant fruit pie may contain as many as 129 calories (51% of the total calories) from fat. Many fast foods are deep fried, which adds additional calories and fat.

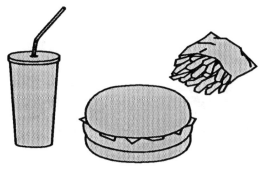

Watch out for Fast Foods !

- **You also need to pay attention to the cholesterol in your diet.** Dietary cholesterol is less important than saturated fat in its effect on your blood cholesterol, but you should still limit foods high in cholesterol. Experts recommend that you eat no more than 300 mg of cholesterol each day. This is not too difficult to achieve. The most concentrated source of dietary cholesterol is the egg yolk. Each yolk contains about 210 mg of cholesterol, so two eggs for breakfast provide you with much more cholesterol than is recommended for that day. You should keep your egg consumption to no more than about four a week. Organ meats, such as liver, also are high in cholesterol, so excessive consumption of these foods is discouraged. This piece of advice is not difficult for most Americans to follow!

A final word about dietary cholesterol. Remember that cholesterol comes **only from animal sources**; plants have no cholesterol. Unscrupulous food processors frequently advertise a product as having no cholesterol. If it comes from plant sources, you can be sure that the statement is true. The catch is that the product may be loaded with fat, and perhaps even saturated fat. In fact, when I see an ad touting a product as "low cholesterol," I assume that it is probably high in fat and should be avoided.

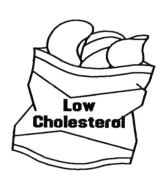

Watch for Deceptive Labels

The few tips presented here on how to follow a nutritionally sound diet are certainly not intended to be a complete discussion of the issues. I have oversimplified to make a few key points, and you should refer to other sources for a more thorough review of the topic. However, you can make a good deal of progress toward a healthy diet by:

— *eating a variety of foods*

— *eating more fruits, vegetables, and whole grains*

— *cutting back on fats, especially saturated fats*.

Don't eat the cheeseburger; have a fruit salad for lunch instead.

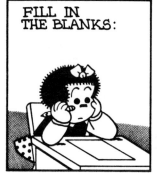
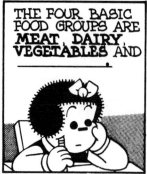
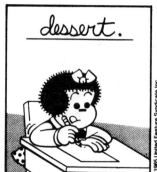
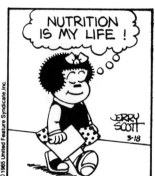

Chapter 6

TAKE IT OFF WITH EXERCISE

INTRODUCTION

Our society is obsessed with thinness. Most of us yearn to look like the models in health club advertisements. About one-half of adult American women and one-quarter of the men report dieting to lose weight. The figure is even higher in teenage girls. Some Yuppie parents restrict the diets of their small infants in an attempt to prevent overweight.

The cause of this preoccupation with dieting and leanness is obscure. It is probably, at least partly, related to the national emphasis on exercise and other healthy lifestyle elements that have received increased attention over the past 25 to 30 years. But it is ironic that health is a driving force behind the diet mania. There is very little evidence that mild overweight causes health problems. I am not, of course, referring to gross obesity or massive overweight. Those conditions are serious medical problems, and individuals who are massively overweight are much more prone to numerous chronic diseases and early death.

Overweight is not a risk factor for early death or death from cardiovascular disease or cancer in our population of patients examined at the Cooper Clinic. Many other studies show similar death rates for lean and mildly overweight persons. The graph below shows mortality ratios for each level of a weight index from more than 750,000 American men and women. The data are from a 12-year follow up of these individuals conducted by Lew and Garfinkel of the American Cancer Society.

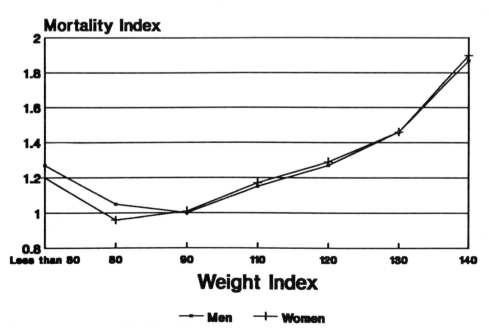

Risk of Death by Weight Index Groups

Source: *Journal of Chronic Disease*, 32: 563-576, 1979.

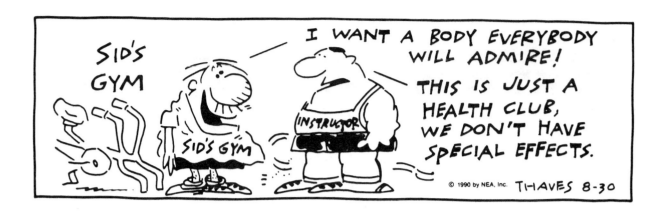

The weight index in this graph was calculated by dividing each person's weight by the average weight for others of the same sex, height, and age and multiplying by 100. Thus, persons of average weight have an index of 100, those below average have an index below 100, and persons heavier than average have a score above 100. Keep in mind that the average adult American is not lean. In this sample, the average man who was 5' 10" tall and weighed about 170-179 pounds. The average 5' 5" woman weighed between 130-139 pounds. These weights are not those of the idealized model or movie star.

The mortality index in the graph shows the relative all-cause death rates for the different weight index groups. Values above 1.0 indicate higher death rates. For example, a mortality index of 1.2 means that persons in that weight index group have a 20% higher death rate than the average-weight men and women.

Death rates are elevated by about 20% in the leanest men and women (those below 80 on the weight index). The lowest death rates (mortality index of 1.0) in this study were observed in men and women between 80 and 110 on the weight index. This range includes about 77% of the men and 74% of the women in the study, so the great majority of the group were not at increased risk of death due to their weight. Risk of death increases substantially at 120 and higher on the weight index, but these groups constitute less than 10% of the total population. A man, 5' 10" tall, would have to weigh more than 200 pounds to be in the 120 weight index group. A women, 5' 5" tall, would have to weigh more than 165 pounds to be in this high risk group.

I offer this information to illustrate that moderate degrees of overweight are not associated with increased risk of major health problems and early death. Most persons who are 10 pounds, or even 20 pounds overweight, do not have increased health risks. In fact, one can probably weigh 30-40 pounds more than the models and still enjoy optimal health.

Even small weight losses

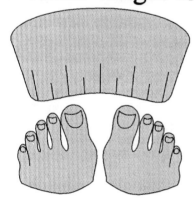

can be beneficial

I must point out that there are some exceptions to this generalization. If you have some other health risk, such as high blood pressure or high cholesterol, even a modest degree of excess body weight may be a problem. Individuals who are a bit plump and have a cholesterol of 240 mg/dl or more should attempt to lose 5 or 10 pounds and check the effect on their cholesterol levels. Small weight losses can be quite beneficial for some individuals.

THE EFFECT OF WEIGHT CYCLING

I discussed earlier the emphasis on thinness and the high percentage of dieting in America. It is apparent that, in spite of continued attempts to lose weight, most people have little success. The U.S. population has gotten progressively heavier during the 20th century. Further evidence of a lack of success with weight loss is the almost weekly appearance of a new diet book on the best seller lists. Most of these books are based on unsound dietary and behavioral theories and practices, and are successful only in the short term, if at all. The most bizarre approach may, however, help produce a temporary loss of a few pounds. But the dieter soon reverts to his or her customary diet, and the lost weight returns. Consequently, there are thousands of men and women, if not millions, whose weight frequently fluctuate.

This frequent weight fluctuation has been viewed by health experts merely as evidence of the failure of diets to produce permanent weight loss. Current research, however, suggests there may be harmful effects associated with this type of weight fluctuation. Recent studies, including our own follow-up of more than 12,000 men over about a four-year period, show higher death rates in individuals whose weights are variable compared to individuals whose weights are stable. In these studies, men and women with a high degree of weight fluctuation were about twice as likely to die during follow-up as those with stable weights. Periodic fluctuations of even 10 pounds appear to increase risk. These research findings are new, and many of the studies are still in progress and have not been published. Although preliminary, these studies should heighten concern about the common yo-yo dieting syndrome.

Avoid YO-YO Dieting

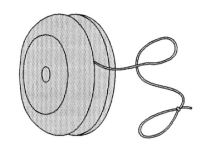

The potential ill effects of yo-yo dieting and the simple fact that most diets are unsuccessful, indicate the importance of a long term approach to weight control. *The LEARN Program for Weight Control* by Kelly D. Brownell, Ph.D., emphasizes a behavioral approach. This book can help you use behaviorally sound methods to control your weight. The LEARN program can also help you make permanent changes in your lifestyle to produce long-term success in weight management. One of the key features of Dr. Brownell's book is the emphasis on increasing physical activity. His recommendations on this point are strongly supported by numerous researchers. For most people who have a weight problem, the probability of long-term success is greatly increased if regular physical activity becomes a key ingredient of the effort.

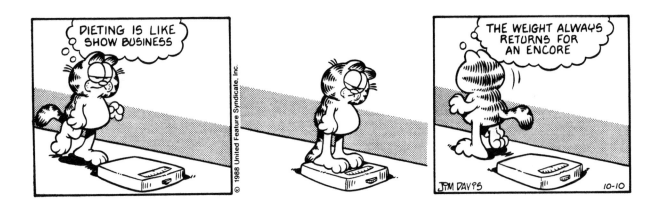

83

THE EFFECT OF EXERCISE
ON WEIGHT REDUCTION

You probably have heard conflicting stories about exercising to lose weight. One friend may swear by exercise as the only way she was able to control her weight. Others may tell you that exercise doesn't help with weight loss because you have to walk an enormous number of miles to lose even one pound, and besides, you will drink one Coke after aerobics class that will replace all of the calories you just burned. In this section, I will present some of the facts about exercise and its effect on body weight regulation. Exercise will not make us all slim, but overall it will help in weight control. I do not want to mislead you, but simply report the state of our knowledge.

First, the bottom line. Exercise **is** an effective way to help control body weight. There have been dozens of controlled exercise training studies conducted over the past 20 years. Many of the studies were conducted very carefully, with random assignments of subjects to exercise or control groups, and with other important scientific design features. Objective laboratory methods were followed to obtain the data, and amount of exercise was precisely regulated with supervised exercise sessions. In virtually all of these studies, the group assigned to exercise, lost weight over the weeks and months they were supervised. The typical average weight loss was in the range of 5 to 10 pounds. Because this is an average, some people lost a good deal more than that; some lost no weight and some actually gained. Usually the gainers did not gain much, and what they gained tended to be muscle or other active tissue, not fat.

There is no precise way to predict who will gain and who will lose weight in an exercise program. But individuals who are lean probably are less likely to lose, because they do not have the fat to lose in the first place! Those who have been quite sedentary and who are relatively lean are the ones who may gain weight with exercise. They have small underdeveloped muscles that will grow with the exercise stimulus. Individuals most likely to lose weight with exercise are those who have been sedentary and are somewhat overweight. Most studies suggest that those who exercise more, lose more weight.

Exercise IS Important for Weight Control

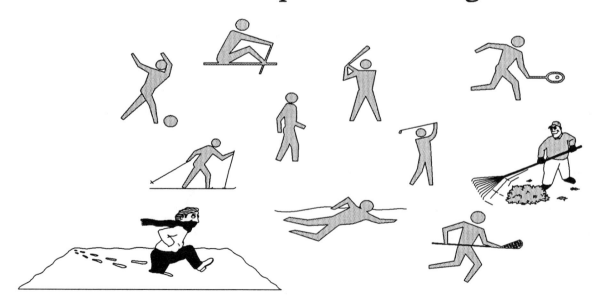

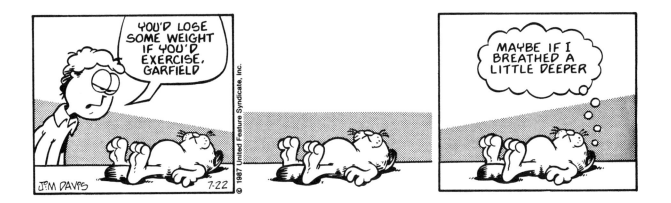

Dramatic differences in body weight are seen in individuals who do a lot of vigorous exercise. In Chapter 5, I briefly described a study we did a few years ago with men and women runners. The 34 men and 27 women were running 35 to 40 miles a week on the average. Although their diets were not qualitatively different from non-exercising community controls, there were large differences in body weights. The men runners weighed almost 25 pounds less than the average U. S. man. The women runners were more than 30 pounds lighter than the average women. A major benefit of exercise for people trying to control their weight is that the effect seems to be more long-lasting than that achieved by dieting alone. Controlled studies do indicate that both diet and exercise are about equally effective in weight loss programs. But most studies, in which dieting alone has been used for weight loss, show that most of the weight is regained within a year or two. As I discussed before, this yo-yo pattern is now thought to be harmful to health. The weight regain, after loss by dieting, is seen even in individuals who have lost large amounts of weight, 40-50 pounds or more. The best success in keeping the weight off seems to occur in individuals who combine exercise with dieting.

Myths about Exercise and Weight Loss

There are many silly and unscientific ideas about the effect of exercise on metabolism, and on weight loss in particular. Many of these have been popularized by best selling books, but a book's success does not insure its accuracy or validity. Several of the more common myths are discussed below.

- *Specific exercises techniques must be used in order to burn the body's fat stores.*
This is one of the most widely held misconceptions about exercise and weight loss. The myth holds that you need to exercise at a specific exercise intensity and for a minimum number of minutes before you burn fat. Part of the misconception stems from the belief that the body either burns carbohydrates or it burns fats. The fact is, most of the time the body is burning both fats and carbohydrates in its metabolic processes. If you are seated at rest while reading this book, you are burning about 1.25 calories a minute (at least for those weighing 150 pounds; if you weigh more or less than 150 pounds, the rate is higher or lower). Approximately one-half of these calories are from fat and one-half from carbohydrate.

The mixture of fuel used for muscular contraction varies under different conditions, but, again, in most instances, both fats and carbohydrates are burned. If you start exercising, the mixture of fuel shifts so that more carbohydrate and less fat is used. At near maximum exercise intensity, the predominate fuel is carbohydrate. When you exercise at a moderate intensity, you first use more carbohydrates than fats. You gradually shift the fuel ratio and use more fats, as the exercise continues for 20 to 30 minutes.

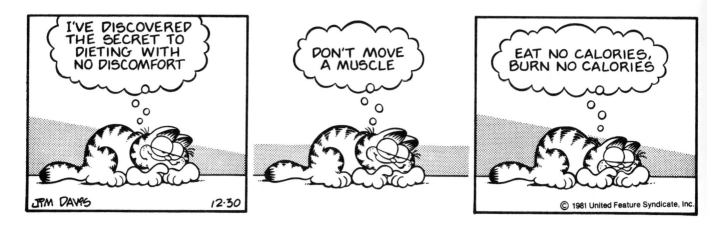

The type of fuel used in varying intensities and durations of exercise was established by carefully controlled experiments in exercise laboratories. The brief review given here is factual. A common problem is that this discussion of fuel use has essentially nothing to do with loss of body fat. You do not have to burn only fat, or even predominately fat, during exercise to lose weight. A calorie burned is a calorie burned, and it doesn't matter whether it was from a fat or a carbohydrate fuel source. There is no evidence I know of that supports the notion that using exercises in which fat is the primary fuel has any beneficial impact on weight control.

The key factor is that if you exercise, you use calories and this helps with weight loss. The more you exercise, the more calories you burn, and the greater the effect on weight reduction.

- *Specific exercises burn fat from specific areas of the body.* It would be wonderful if specific exercises could be used to remove fat from a particular location. Unfortunately, it just isn't possible. Most exercise books and articles present exercises "for your hips" or "for your abdomen" or some other part of your body. The implication is that you merely have to identify your fat deposits and design a specific set of exercises to remove them. But that doesn't happen. Specific exercises can strengthen specific muscles or increase flexibility around a joint used in the activity, or burn calories and contribute to overall weight control in that way. They do not slim or spot-reduce hips or thighs.

- *Exercise increases your resting metabolism.* This is another idea that sounds good, and it would be great if it were true. The concept is that your metabolic rate remains elevated for an extended time after your exercise session, or is permanently set at a higher level. You are supposed to get a double benefit from your workout; you expend energy while exercising, and continue to burn calories at a faster rate for several hours after the session ends.

It does take some time before your metabolic rate returns to baseline. In fact, if you do an exhausting bout of exercise, it may take 30 minutes to an hour before your energy expenditure is back to where it was before the exercise. This is due to the "paying back" of an oxygen deficit created by the exhausting exercise, and to the effect of elevated body temperature on metabolic rate. There are a few studies that suggest energy expenditure remains slightly elevated for several hours after exercise, but other studies show no effect. If there is some slight increase in energy metabolism for several hours, the total effect on caloric balance would be minimal.

- *Does regular exercise cause a relatively permanent increase in resting metabolism?* Can you get in shape and have your body function like a little furnace and burn calories at a high rate? Probably not. If fit individuals have a higher resting energy expenditure, it is most likely due to their having a greater muscle mass; muscle is metabolically active. The studies on this point are inconclusive. Once again, the greatest value of exercise in a weight control program is in the calories burned in the actual exercise. Rather than relying on a slight increase

86

in caloric expenditure for an extended time after exercise, you would be better off simply walking for another minute or so.

- **You cannot burn many calories by exercise; you have to run 35 miles to lose one pound.** The second half of this statement is correct. One pound of body fat yields about 3,500 calories. A person who weighs 150 pounds will burn about 100 calories walking or running one mile. So if you wanted to burn the caloric equivalent of one pound of body fat by walking, you would have to cover 35 miles. It is unlikely that anyone will attempt to do this, at least in one exercise session. But you do not have to do it at one time. If you walked or ran five miles a day, you would cover 35 miles in a week. And the effect on weight loss should be comparable.

The problem is that you do not want to only lose one pound a week. We expect or maybe demand instant results. But it just doesn't happen that way. You did not put the excess weight on quickly. It also takes 3,500 extra calories to add a pound of body fat. It would be very difficult to consume that many calories above your caloric requirement in a short time. You accumulated the weight you now want to lose by eating a few additional calories at a time, and the result was the extra fat that appeared over a period of weeks, months or years.

I recommend that you take a gradual approach to getting enough exercise to assist with weight control. Follow the advice given in earlier chapters about building exercise into your life at every opportunity. And remember, it will take more exercise to have a significant impact on body weight than it will to affect your fitness or improve your health status. I believe the best way to use exercise in a weight control program is to build up to an hour a day of moderate exercise. Brisk walking is fine. I do not know if the effect of 30 two-minute walks a day will have the same effect on weight loss as a one-hour walk, but I do believe it is reasonable to begin your exercise program for weight control by accumulating multiple small bouts of exercise each day. This will help get you into the habit of doing exercise, burn calories, improve your fitness, and make a contribution to your health. If weight control is one of your main exercise objectives, I suspect that you will make more progress if you make your brisk walks 30 minutes to an hour long, and try to get at least one hour in each day.

You also should combine your exercise program with modest caloric restriction. If you exercise 500 calories a day and reduce your dietary intake by 500 calories a day, you would have a caloric deficit of 7,000 calories a week. This is comparable to two pounds of fat, and is the maximum weekly rate of weight loss recommended by the experts.

Recommendations:

1. Take the gradual approach to accumulating sufficient exercise to assist with weight control.

2. Build up to an hour a day of moderate exercise.

3. Combine your exercise program with modest caloric restriction.

I must caution against taking too literally a mathematical approach to determining weight loss. The human body is an intricate and complex machine, and many other factors effect energy balance and weight control. When you begin to manipulate diet and exercise to create a deficit of calories, your body responds by shutting down the metabolic rate. Your energy expenditure at rest and during moderate exercise may be reduced by 10 to 20 percent. This is why it is so hard to lose weight. The body is trying to preserve its mass. This probably is an evolutionary response that had survival value for our ancient ancestors. In times of famine, reducing energy expenditure to preserve the body mass was important. Unfortunately, in our society, with abundant and inexpensive food readily available, it is not needed. And, in fact, it has adverse effects on attempts to lose weight.

You may not be able to strictly regulate energy intake and expenditure and precisely estimate your rate of weight loss. This should not discourage you from changing your exercising and eating habits to establish a negative caloric balance and gradually produce weight loss.

Advantages of Exercise in Weight Control

Weight control is a difficult process for many individuals. Our society seems to conspire against our efforts to lose and maintain weight. Food is cheap and plentiful, we have many labor-saving devices available to us, and many pleasurable sedentary activities to enjoy. Exercise is not a cure-all for overweight, but regular exercise can be useful in many ways in your weight control program.

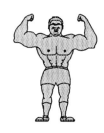

- **Exercise tends to build muscle tissue.** This has many benefits. Muscle cells are metabolically active and they burn more calories in basal metabolism than do fat cells. Thus, the more muscle you have, the more energy you burn while at rest. Weight lost by dieting tends to come from both body fat stores and from muscles. So in this circumstance, you lose functional tissue along with the fat and also **reduce** your resting metabolic requirement.

- **Exercise is a proactive behavior.** Unlike dieting, where you are cutting something out, exercise is adding a desirable habit. Because there are many benefits to exercising, you should feel that you are achieving something beyond weight control. You are doing something for yourself.

As I stated earlier, individuals who exercise more adjust their intake of calories to a higher level. The increased energy needed for exercise ultimately has to come from food. However, people who exercise a lot are leaner, so exercise must help regulate their appetites. Also, as mentioned in Chapter 5, there is another benefit of exercise relative to appetite control. Exercise appears to temporarily blunt the appetite. If you feel hungry, try a bout of exercise. First of all, you are not likely to eat while exercising. You will probably find that your hunger pangs have passed, and may not return for an hour or two.

I discussed earlier the body mass-sparing mechanism that is activated when you begin to diet. When you establish a deficit of calories, your body begins to shut down its metabolic processes. The rate at which you burn calories at rest and the energy cost of moderate intensity, exercise may be reduced by 20% or more. This mechanism tends to defeat the purpose of dieting. More research is needed, but preliminary studies suggest that exercise may prevent, or at least reduce, this decline in the body's metabolism.

Several studies over the past 10 to 15 years show that exercise, behavioral modification dietary programs, and combinations of diet and exercise, have about the same short term effect of weight loss. Studies over 10 to 20 weeks show approximately equal reductions in weight for these separate conditions. When the study subjects are followed for one or two years in the maintenance phase of the program, striking differences emerge. The typical study shows that individuals who lost weight by dieting alone gain most of the weight back after a year. Individuals who used exercise, either alone or in combination with diet, are much more likely to have maintained a weight loss during a long-term follow up. This same finding is now reported for individuals who lose large amounts of weight in very low-calorie, medically monitored, liquid diet programs. For such an individual, who usually has lost very large amounts of weight, long-term maintenance of weight loss is much more likely if the person has established a regular exercise program.

Long-term maintenance of weight loss is much more likely if a regular exercise program has been established.

SUMMARY

Overweight is a problem for millions of Americans. It is difficult for many individuals to lose weight and to maintain their goal weight. The best strategy appears to be a combination of caloric restriction and an increase in exercise. The problem must be approached from a long-term behavioral change perspective for optimal success. Dr. Brownell's *The LEARN Program for Weight Control* provides considerable information about techniques for behavioral weight control. It can be used with this book to structure an exercise and diet program for optimal weight control.

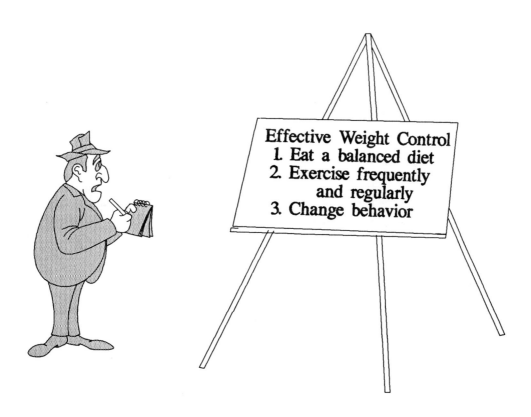

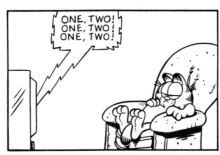

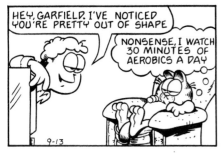

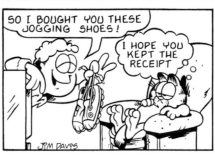

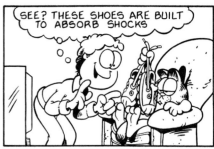

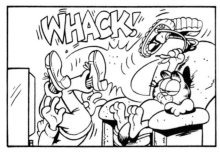

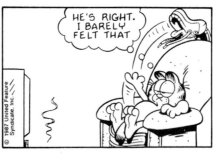

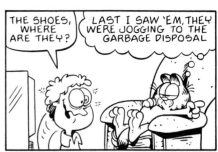

Chapter 7

KEEP IT UP

In previous chapters, I have suggested ways on how to start increasing your physical activity. I have emphasized a step-by-step approach to altering your exercise behavior. I hope you have analyzed carefully your attitudes and beliefs about exercise and have begun to make changes. If you are now routinely building in more opportunities to be active and have specifically planned a few two- or three-minute walks each day, you should be ready to take the next step. As always, it is important to build slowly on previous success. Try to avoid rushing the process. If you are still having difficulty making changes, go back to the previous chapters and revise your earlier plans.

If you have already adopted some new exercise behaviors, you are now ready to move forward.

THE FIVE-MINUTE WALK

The Five-Minute Walk

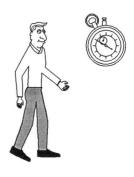

Perhaps you saw this coming. I have tried to get you started with a simple two-minute walk. Now, I am jumping to five minutes. Is that fair? More than doubling the time may be an intolerable burden. How can a busy person who has many responsibilities, possibly find those extra three minutes? Well, of course, I am being sarcastic. I do not intend to ask you to do the impossible. I am firmly committed to the principle that making behavioral changes in small increments is the best approach for most individuals. If increasing from two or three minutes of walking to five minutes in a single session, proves difficult for you right now, simply continue with your previous plan. Perhaps you may wish to revise it and build in a few more short walks before lengthening the time of some of the walks.

Take heart. I am not going to try to get you up to one-hour walks, although that would be fine too. I think that an appropriate minimum target to consider is three to four 10-minute walks a day (or the equivalent). Later in the book, I will suggest that you add such walks to your day. This amount of exercise will get you into the moderate fitness group described in Chapter 1. Remember that the men and women in our study who had at least moderate levels of fitness had much lower death rates than the less fit men and women. I still endorse the idea that **even some exercise is better than none.** I believe that setting the moderate fitness level as a goal is reasonable and will almost certainly provide important health and functional benefits.

How Can I Fit in a Five-Minute Walk?

How can you increase some of the two- or three-minute walks to five minutes? I suggest that you review how and when you have been able to fit the two minute walks into your day. Analyze your schedule and determine which ones can be extended with minimal disruption to your other activities. For example, suppose that you have been taking a two minute walk as soon as you get up in the morning. Surely you can extend for three more minutes. If your morning schedule is so rushed that you do not have any additional time at all, reset your alarm clock five minutes earlier.

IT'S NOT SO BAD

Early in the morning, as the alarm goes off at five,

the sound is so annoying. But my body, I cannot deprive,

I must get out of bed, for there is no way to improvise,

for now I have adapted to a life of exercise.

My feet pound along the pavement, just at the break of dawn,

but to my amazement, I feel great as the day goes on.

Ann Blair

Do you watch any television? If so, you can squeeze in a five-minute walk between programs. The sign-off credits, commercials, and opening scenes of the next program usually take at least five minutes. Use that opportunity to take a quick walk around the block. Or, if you live in a high-rise building, use the time for five minutes of stair climbing.

Are you taking a two- or three-minute walk at lunchtime? It should be relatively easy to extend it to five minutes. Perhaps you can take a five-minute walk at the start of your lunch hour, and take another one at the end. Do that and you will have almost one-third of the daily exercise dose that will get you into the moderate fitness category.

There are obviously many ways and times into which you can squeeze a five-minute walk. Use your creativity. Find out what will work for you. At this point, you do not need to extend all of your shorter walks to five minutes, but I suggest you plan to extend at least one or two of them each day. Give the idea some serious thought and list on the following chart how you can take at least one five-minute walk.

Ways to Increase Your Walking Time

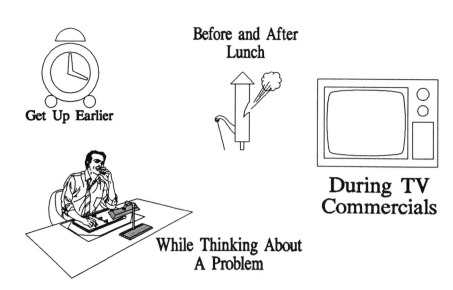

Get Up Earlier

Before and After Lunch

During TV Commercials

While Thinking About A Problem

```
┌─────────────────────────────────────────────────────────────────────┐
│                  My Plans for Five-Minute Walks                       │
│    1. _____         │
│                                                                       │
│    2. _____         │
│                                                                       │
│    3. _____         │
│                                                                       │
│    4. _____         │
│                                                                       │
│    5. _____         │
│                                                                       │
│    Next week, I will attempt to take _____ five-minute walks each day. │
└─────────────────────────────────────────────────────────────────────┘
```

WHAT GOOD IS THE FIVE-MINUTE WALK DOING

Trust me, I am really not trying to trick you. One or two five-minute walks a day and two or three shorter walks will not make you highly fit. It will be enough exercise to begin to make an impact if you are a sedentary individual. We need more research to specifically document the physiological effects of short bouts of moderate exercise, but I am convinced that even the small dose of exercise discussed here may have benefits. For instance, it does not appear to take a great deal of exercise to reduce blood clotting ability. Getting up early for a few minutes of brisk walking may be sufficient.

A few minutes of brisk walking may also lower blood pressure for an hour or two. This is not a permanent reduction, but a temporary effect. It may well have health benefits, especially for those with elevated blood pressures. Several walks during the day could result in several hours of lower blood pressure.

Also, climbing a few flights of stairs may help strengthen leg muscles. There is some evidence that weight-bearing activity, such as walking and stair climbing, may have other musculoskeletal benefits, such as increasing bone strength.

The accumulative effect of several short exercise sessions can result in significant increases in the number of calories you burn. Remember that brisk walking increases caloric expenditure three to fourfold, while stair climbing may increase expenditure by up to 10 times or more. Thirty minutes of brisk walking accumulated over a day would result in an increase in expenditure of about 150 calories for a 150-pound person. That does not seem like very much, but continued day after day, it can add up to an impressive total. An extra 150 calories a day becomes 1,050 calories a week, more than 4,000 a month, and almost 55,000 calories a year. That is the energy equivalent of more than 15 pounds of fat in a year.

Now don't misunderstand; I am not saying that you will lose 15 pounds in a year. As discussed earlier, weight control is an extremely complex metabolic process, and we invariably overestimate the weight loss impact of diet and exercise. But the basic point remains; you can accumulate impressive totals of calories burned from repeated short exercise sessions. The overall effect on weight control will be beneficial.

I do not claim that a five-minute walk will extend your life, make you rich and successful, and insure good social relationships. The research evidence does, however, support the conclusion that moderate amounts of exercise and fitness have major health benefits. Behavioral science research also supports the notion that building health habit change in small increments is the surest way to long-term success. When you get to the point of one or two five-minute walks a day, plus a few other shorter bouts of walking or other activities, you are well on your way to establishing new habits, and have improved your health.

DEVELOPING AND MAINTAINING SUPPORT

Social support is an important ingredient in the behavioral change process. You are more likely to be successful if your family, friends, and co-workers are supportive than if they actively oppose, or are even indifferent to your efforts toward change. Social support can occur in many forms. It may be nothing more than encouragement and reinforcement of your attempts to change your exercise habits. Or, people who wish to support your efforts might offer specific rewards or exercise with you. Some support is likely to occur naturally as those around you notice that you are working on increasing your exercise. You can generate support by doing some specific planning. A few suggestions follow.

Gather Social Support

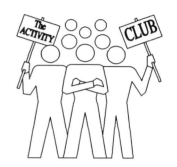

Spouse or Partner Support

Your spouse or living partner is likely to be one of the most significant persons in your life. He or she can have an important impact on your attempts to adopt new exercise habits. If your partner complains about what you are doing, or tries to sabotage your plans, it will be difficult for you to succeed. Active encouragement and support from your partner will increase your likelihood of success.

An exercise break with your spouse or partner is an excellent opportunity for some high-quality communication. My wife and I are both runners, and some of our best discussions and problem-solving sessions have occurred while running. Ask your spouse or partner to join you on some of your walks or other exercise sessions. Discuss the events of the day, family issues, or the news. You may find that your relationship is strengthened.

Ask your spouse or partner to provide appropriate reinforcement for your exercise habit changes. He or she does not have to go overboard, but recognition will make you feel good, and increase the chances that you will continue the activity.

Spouse or Partner Support

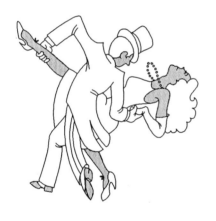

Children

Do you have children or grandchildren? Look for opportunities to play with them, take a walk, or engage in some other activity. Take them to the zoo or on some other outing that requires walking, hiking, or some other activity. This will provide a good opportunity to talk and find out about their feelings and thoughts. It also serves as a good example to them that exercise is fun and important.

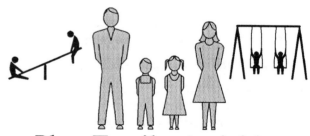

Plan Family Activities

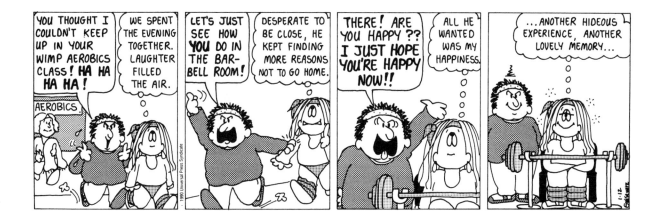

Friends or Neighbors

Some people find that it is easier to make exercise changes if they make a commitment to another person. Arrange to take your early morning walk with a neighbor. If you know that someone is waiting for you, you are more likely to get out of bed and go exercise. Otherwise it is too easy to roll over and go back to sleep with the promise to yourself that you will make it up tomorrow. Meet a friend at lunch time and walk to a favorite restaurant. You will enjoy the visit and the pleasure will reinforce your exercise.

CASE EXAMPLE

Role Model for Exercise

We are influenced by those around us, especially by persons we admire. Many of the habits and characteristics you have are likely to be due partly to your parents, a former teacher, a neighbor, friend, or co-worker. Do you have someone you admire because of their exercise habits? I am not referring to a star athlete, such as Florence Griffith Joyner or Bo Jackson. Let's face it. You are not likely to ever have a body that looks like that, and you certainly are not going to be that fast or strong.

Rather, do you have a friend, neighbor, or family member whom you look up to who has established a regular exercise program? Maybe your grandmother walks every day even though she is somewhat feeble and has arthritis. Perhaps a friend who is nonathletic and had been sedentary for years has started running and completed a 10K race. Talk to these people about how and why they established a regular program of exercise. Use them as role models. If they can do it, so can you.

Join a Walking Club

Walking is becoming a favorite form of exercise for many people. This popularity has led to several organizations that can be helpful in providing motivation and social support. There are several walking clubs, newsletters, books, and magazines. Information about walking can provide an exerciser with beneficial information. On the next page is a list of resources for walkers. You may also want to check the weekend section of your local newspapers for walking events sponsored by local walking clubs.

Resources for Walkers

American Volksport Association
1001 Pat Booker Road, Suite 203
Universal City, TX 78148
(512) 659-2112

Can send you a list of walking clubs in your area. Publishes *American Wanderer* $12 per yr. subscription ($8 bulk rate).

Prevention Walking Club
Rodale Press
Box 6099
Emmaus, PA 18099
(800) 441-7761

Quarterly newsletter and annual magazine dealing with all aspects of walking.
Membership cost is $9.97 per year.

Rockport Walking Institute
P.O. Box 480
Marlboro, MA 01752
(508) 485-2090 (ext. 114)

Will send educational materials on fitness walking, diet and exercise. Call or send self-addressed, business-sized envelope with $.58 postage affixed.

Walkabout International
835 Fifth Avenue, Room 407
San Diego, CA 92101
(619) 231-SHOE

Club with chapters in various cities. Organizes & publishes information about walks.

WalkWays Center
733 15th Street, NW
Washington, DC 20005
(202) 737-9555

Non-profit clearinghouse for information on aspects of walking. Publishes a newsletter (*Walkways Almanac*) 8 times per year; $17 for one year, $29 for two years.

Walking Inc.
9-11 Harcourt St.
Boston, MA 02116
(617) 266-3322

Bi-monthly commercial magazine about walking. $12 per year for subscription.

STRUCTURING YOUR SUPPORT NETWORK

The few suggestions above are intended to serve as examples to stimulate your thinking. How can you generate and maintain social support for your new exercise habits? On the next page, jot down a few ways.

DEALING WITH RELAPSE

No matter how good your intentions and how carefully you develop your plans to increase your exercise, you will occasionally have difficulty making changes. Behavioral psychologists call this relapse. You may make changes and be doing well until something happens to interfere with your new program. You may get sick or take an extended business trip. You and your family may go on vacation. You may have company or get quite busy at work. You can be certain that disruptions to your schedule will occur. But they do not have to permanently destroy your new exercise habits. Many problems can be avoided by proper planning.

If you are going on a business trip, think in advance about how you will maintain your physical activity level. If you have a favorite pair of walking shoes, be sure to pack them. If rope jumping is your thing, be sure you take your rope. Convince yourself that the trip will not cause you to stop exercising. I actually find that I tend to do more running when I travel. When you are on a trip, you are freed of some of your usual responsibilities at home and work, and may have more discretionary time than when you are at home. Also, nothing is better for relaxation after a long meeting or a hard day on the road than a run or a long walk.

Vacations offer many excellent opportunities for increasing your exercise. The best way to see the sights in a new city is to get a map and take a walking tour. Hiking a country or mountain trail can be a terrific experience. Consider your vacation a chance to enjoy a new or familiar recreational activity. I have

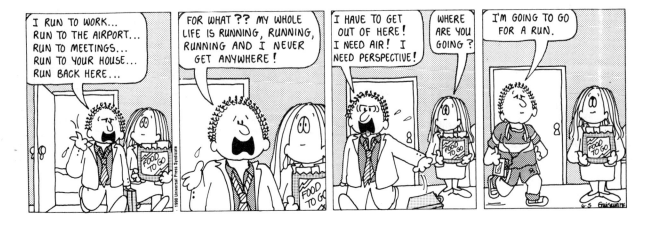

97

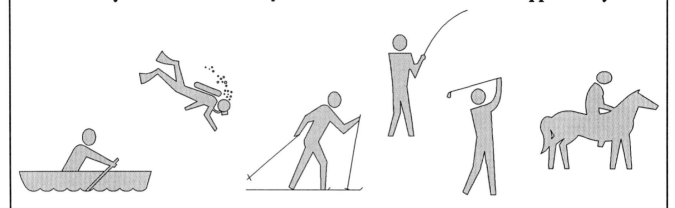

What do you like to do that you don't often have time and opportunity for?

Build these activities into your next vacation !

only been snorkeling four or five times, but I plan to do it again whenever I can. Cross-country skiing is not big in Dallas, so I look forward for the chance to go to a location where it is possible. What do you like to do that you don't often have the time or the opportunity to do? Is there some new activity that you have always wanted to try? Build these activities into your next vacation.

You will occasionally get sick or have an injury that precludes exercise. Do not let this be an excuse to stop permanently. Plan for exercise and normal activities to be resumed, and set the date when you will start again. You may have to go back through some of the earlier methods you used to get started, and you may have to reduce the amount of exercise for a few days or a couple of weeks, but strive to get back on your schedule.

If your family realizes that regular activity is now part of your routine and is important to you, they will be able to help you stay on schedule. When our children were younger, it was sometimes hard to find time for exercise. Once, when I was out of town and unable to babysit, my wife was having difficulty finding time to run. After a few days, she said, "I guess I'll just stop running. It is too hard to find the time." Our daughter, who was three at the time, said, "But, Mommy, what about your health?" That gave Jane the encouragement to juggle her schedule to make time for exercise.

Disruptions to your exercise plans will occur. Expect them and plan how you will overcome these types of circumstances as soon as possible. You should be thinking of yourself now as a person who is a regular exerciser. That is your natural status. After temporary disruptions in your exercise schedule, work diligently to get back on track.

After Temporary Disruptions, Get Back on Track

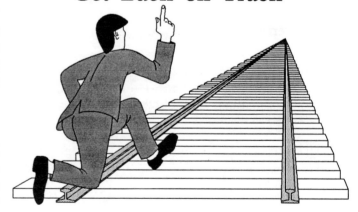

Chapter 8

EXERCISE AND FITNESS IN CHILDREN AND YOUTH

Are you concerned about your children's fitness? Does it seem that America's children and youth are sedentary and overweight? What should be done about the problem? I will discuss these and other questions in this chapter and suggest what you can do to help your children maintain an active lifestyle.

ARE U.S. CHILDREN AND YOUTH ACTIVE AND FIT

Your answer to the question in the heading above is probably "no." Most people seem to believe that children and youth are quite inactive and have low levels of physical fitness. The answer to this question is not simple, and it is not entirely clear what answer is correct. I do not agree that most of our young people are unfit, but there is some cause for concern.

Fitness Propaganda

In the mid-1950s, researchers from Columbia University published reports indicating that American students were more likely to fail a simple physical fitness test than students in several European countries. This finding came to the attention of President Eisenhower, and he became concerned about the apparent problem. His reaction was to form the forerunner of today's President's Council on Physical Fitness and Sports.

The message from that Council and physical educators has been unrelenting for the past 35 years. The status of youth fitness has been lamented and a crisis proclaimed. This point of view has been accepted uncritically, and almost everyone I ask believes that most American children are unfit. Few people stop to think about the quality of the data and the soundness of the reasoning that leads to this conclusion. A few facts may help put the issue into perspective:

- The test used in the research to compare American and European children was a test of minimum muscular fitness. There were several items, all scored as pass or fail. For example, one test was to do one push-up; another was to bend forward and touch the toes while keeping the knees straight. If students failed one item, they failed the entire test. American children were much more likely than European children to fail the flexibility item. Thus, the youth fitness crisis was primarily based on the failure of children in the study to touch their toes!

- The reaction of physical educators to this perceived problem was to develop and implement a youth fitness test. Ironically, the tests used up until 1980 did not include a test of flexibility.

- One of the stated, primary concerns about the low level of youth fitness was the presumed effect of low fitness on health, especially heart disease. Paradoxically, the tests used to determine children's level of fitness were comprised of items that measured speed or power, such as the 50-yard dash or standing long jump. These items measure an ability that is essential to success in many sports, but it has nothing to do with health.

99

Some Fitness Tests Measure

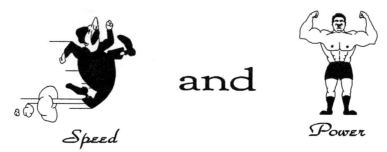

Speed   and   Power

But Do Not Measure

Health-Related Physical Fitness

- Until recently, the experts did not define what an acceptable level of physical fitness was. Large groups of children were evaluated. The experts then published norms from these studies and said, "Isn't it terrible how unfit our children are?" The more important questions are "How much fitness is needed?" and "How many children meet that standard?" This failure to specify fitness standards led to some ridiculous statements. Joseph Califano, when he was secretary of Health, Education and Welfare, was quoted as saying that, "29 million adolescents are unfit." That sounds terrible, but it seems unlikely when you consider that there are only about 29 million adolescents in the entire country. Surely, they are not all unfit. But that is the type of hyperbole we have been subjected to regarding the fitness of our youth.

- Another problem with most of the youth fitness tests used for the past 35 years is the test items. Specific tests included the 50-yard (or meter) dash, the standing long jump, and a shuttle run in which students dashed back and forth between two lines 30 feet apart. These test items measure leg power or speed. As mentioned earlier, this characteristic is important, if not essential, to success in many sports. Speed is unrelated to health or to usual daily activities. Also, speed is primarily genetically determined and cannot be changed appreciably by training. Yet, over the years, millions of American students have been labeled as unfit simply because they did poorly on athletic fitness test items that required speed. A fitness test that emphasized health-related fitness items (cardiorespiratory endurance, body composition, and the like) did become available for national distribution in 1980. Not all fitness professionals agree with this change in focus, however, and acceptance has been slow.

- The use of physical fitness awards for students, further illustrates the muddled thinking of the fitness establishment. The primary award given for many years has been the Presidential Physical Fitness Award. This award was given by the President's Council on Physical Fitness and Sports to students who scored at or above the 85th percentile on all six test items of the American Alliance for Health, Physical Education, Recreation, and Dance's Youth Fitness Test. Since students had to meet the standards on all items, only 2 or 3 percent were able to qualify for the award. Furthermore, the test emphasized speed (as discussed above), so the award winners were the genetically gifted who had been born fast. The implicit message to the vast majority of students who could not win the award, no matter how much they trained or how hard they tried, was that they were not fit.

Fortunately, there are now more reasonable alternatives available for youth fitness programs. My own institution, the Institute for Aerobics Research, has distributed a FITNESSGRAM nationally for the past several years. FITNESSGRAM consists of a health-related physical fitness test. It incorporates an award system based on achieving appropriate exercise behaviors and meeting attainable health fitness standards and includes an educational program for teachers. A teacher administers the fitness test, enters the data into a personal computer, and prints the FITNESSGRAM. The FITNESSGRAM is a computer-report showing the student's achievement on each of the test items, the health standard for each item, and brief messages on how to help the student improve performance on items for which he or she didn't meet the standards.

Several awards are offered by the FITNESSGRAM program. The "Get Fit" award is given to students who complete a six-week physical activity program. This can be done in school or at home. All students can win this award by completing the exercise log indicating that they have participated in the training program. The purpose is to reinforce appropriate exercise habits.

The "I'm Fit" award is given to students who meet the health standards on four of the five test items. The standards were set by the FITNESSGRAM Scientific Advisory Board. These nationally recognized scientists reviewed existing research on exercise, fitness, and health and established fitness standards that are appropriate for a healthy and productive life. At the Institute, we have analyzed FITNESSGRAM test data from more than 30,000 boys and girls and find that most students can meet the health standards. For most items, 70 to 80 percent achieve the standard, and 50 to 60 percent qualify for the "I'm Fit" award. These high award rates are counter to the view that the fitness status of American children and youth is terrible. We really should not be surprised by these results. Children and youth are the most active and fit segment of our society, as anyone who has reared children can assert.

Another FITNESSGRAM award is called "Fit for Life." This award is designed to recognize individuals who have participated in a personal exercise program. "Fit for Life" is for use by families and is appropriate for both parents and children. Participants in this award program record their physical activity on an exercise log. Points are given for participation, based on the type and amount of activity. Awards are won by accumulating activity points, and a wide variety of awards are available. This system can be used to encourage family physical activity. If you are interested in participating, you may obtain the information and free exercise log forms from:

Division of Youth Fitness
Institute for Aerobics Research
12330 Preston Road
Dallas, Texas 75230

You may also contact us at this address if you are interested in getting information about how schools in your community can enroll in FITNESSGRAM.

FITNESSGRAM

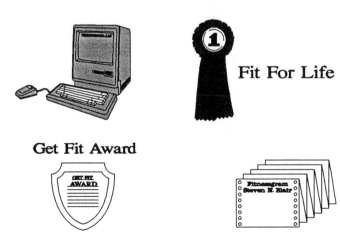

Fit For Life

Get Fit Award

WHAT CAN I DO ABOUT MY CHILD'S PHYSICAL FITNESS

There are several steps you can take to help your children and the children in your community develop and maintain physical fitness, develop a positive attitude about exercise, and establish the habit of regular physical activity. The primary goal probably should not be to force children to engage in vigorous exercise in an attempt to develop a high level of fitness. Most children are already adequately fit. The emphasis should be placed on structuring children's activities to include some active recreation and play, making it fun, encouraging family participation, and establishing the exercise habit.

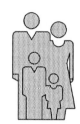

What Can I Do About My Child's Physical Fitness?

Home Activities

For parents, one objective should be to limit the amount of time their children spend in very sedentary activities. All of us need balance in our lives, and children are no exception. A variety of activities is desirable. Children need to be exposed to many opportunities and activities such as active games, sports, reading, and other quiet pastimes; video games, cultural activities, and other things of interest. The average American child probably spends more time watching television than in any other activity. There is nothing inherently bad about watching television, but time spent watching television is time that cannot be spent in active play. Research shows that many children virtually go into a trance while watching television, and their energy expenditure drops.

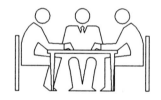
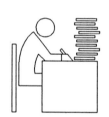
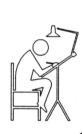

Limit the Amount
of Time You
and Your Family
Spend in
Sedentary Activities

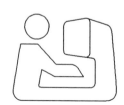

Many Fun Recreational Activities Can Significantly Increase Energy Expenditure For All Family Members

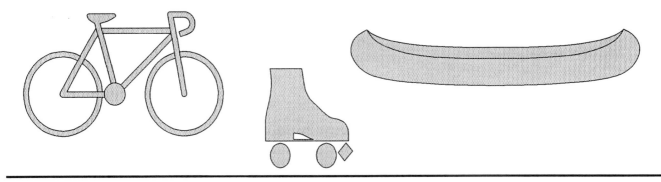

Dr. William Dietz, of Harvard University, has studied the relationship between hours of television viewing each day and obesity in more than 6,000 12- to 17-year-old adolescents. The sample was from the National Health Examination Survey conducted by the National Center for Health Statistics during 1966 to 1970. The percentage of children found to be obese increased by 2% for each hour of television watched per day.

These data are now more than 20 years old, and perhaps it is different today. Yet, somehow I doubt that American adolescents are watching less television. Encourage your children to restrict the amount of very sedentary activities such as television; substitute games, family outings, or other activities that require more energy expenditure.

One excellent way to help your children be more active is to take family outings that promote energy expenditure. Young children will be spontaneously active if you take them to an attractive playground, especially if other children are present. A trip to the zoo or nature center will keep the whole family moving. Many fun recreational activities can significantly increase energy expenditure for all family members. Go roller skating, take a hike, use the bicycle trails in your community for exploring, and enjoy an afternoon rowing or canoeing.

Try to make time each day for some activity with your child. "Walk and talk" as a regular habit will have many benefits. It will give you a chance to discuss your child's feelings, school events, and other matters. If it is not too far, you might walk your child to school instead of driving. It will do you both good and will provide time alone for special talks.

Be a good role model. Communicate to your children that your family you should always be looking for opportunities to be active. Walk instead of drive on short trips, make family gardening or household chores an opportunity to burn calories, and plan for active sports or games.

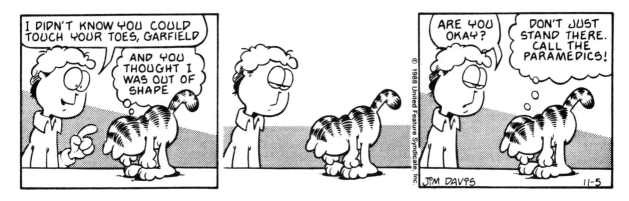

School Activities

Many parents believe that school physical education programs provide for their children's physical activity needs. This may not be true. School physical education programs tend to focus on teaching sports, not concepts of exercise and physical fitness. Recent surveys show that children get the majority of their exercise outside of school, and there is little evidence that physical education programs improve physical fitness. Thus, as parents, you cannot rely on the schools to meet their children's physical fitness needs. I recommend that you consider several points to ensure that your children get enough exercise, develop and maintain fitness, and gain knowledge and attitudes about the importance of exercise and fitness throughout life. Here are some things you can do:

- *First, check with your children's physical education teacher to determine the type of program offered.* If there is an inadequate emphasis on fitness principles and activities, and on teaching about the lifetime value of exercise and fitness, you may want to consider requesting that the school change its program. This can be sensitive and difficult, but if properly approached, schools can be encouraged to make changes.

  Unfortunately, some physical education programs have taught children to dislike physical activity. Using activity as punishment, making fun of the unskilled, and approaching physical education as a Marine boot camp have no place in a modern physical education program. The environment should be supportive and caring and should help children develop a love for activity. What type of physical education program does you child's school have?

- *What type of physical fitness test is used in your children's school?* If the school is using the old type of test that emphasizes speed or power (items such as the 50-meter dash or standing long jump), make the teachers aware of the more modern tests such as FITNESSGRAM. Explain why you think a fitness program should emphasize health-related fitness, rather than athletic fitness, and why health standards for test items are desirable. Discuss how awards recognizing appropriate exercise behavior, that can be won by most children, are preferable to awards that go mostly to elite athletes.

- *Work with schools and other community agencies to provide increased opportunities for active recreation and sports for children.* The more popular sports, such as football, soccer, baseball, and basketball may already be widely available in your area; but other opportunities, especially for individual and noncompetitive activities that can be accomplished throughout life, are usually less common. Try to make your community an active one. Encourage trails for transportation by bicycle or on foot. Make the use of an automobile less convenient for short trips.

SUMMARY

You have the responsibility for your children's physical fitness just as you have for other areas of their development. Help them maintain the spontaneously active habits of childhood. Set a good example and foster attitudes that will help them be active and fit throughout their lives. It is important to their health.

Chapter 9

THE FINAL TOUCH

You have been working on changing your physical activity level for several weeks. You conducted a thorough analysis of your beliefs and attitudes about the value of exercise and made a commitment to change. Most of you made small changes, built on successes, and gradually achieved a consistent exercise habit. Many of you are already exercising at a level that will improve your function and health, but some probably need to make a few more changes to achieve an acceptable exercise level. In this chapter, I will give you some additional tips on how to increase your energy expenditure and how to maintain these new behaviors for the long term.

THE TEN-MINUTE WALK

The Ten-Minute Walk

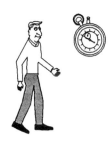

You should now be incorporating several two- to three-minute walks into your daily activities. In the past few weeks, you may have also added a couple of five-minute walks into your routine. You need to maintain many of these habits, but I now recommend that you either add one or two ten-minute walks or extend some of the shorter sessions to ten minutes. I hope that the two-minute walks (or two-minute bouts of stair climbing or other comparable activity) have become so ingrained into your daily routine that you do them almost without thinking. These activities should become a permanent part of your lifestyle.

CHANGING HABITS

Establish the Exercise Habit

I'll bet that most of you brush your teeth at least a couple of times a day. If you are on a trip and forget your toothbrush, you really don't feel right until you get another one and brush, right? Regular brushing is such a well-established habit that you find it almost impossible not to do it. Well, suppose I were to tell you that regular brushing had nothing whatsoever to do with preventing cavities? Would you stop? What if it were shown that brushing actually caused cavities? Would that convince you to throw away your toothbrush? My guess is that even if you were persuaded that brushing was bad for your teeth, you would find it difficult to stop.

Make Regular Exercise
Another Well-Established Habit.

Can you make regular exercise such a well-established habit that you don't feel right if you miss more than a day or two? The answer is yes, and many people have. Some critics have termed this need for exercise an addiction and see it as pathological. I disagree. Some of us, over time, simply become used to regular exercise, just as we do to brushing our teeth. Of course, it is possible to become compulsive about anything, and I suppose that some people are compulsive about exercise. I do not think that one should be neurotic about it, but having a well-ingrained exercise habit is positive.

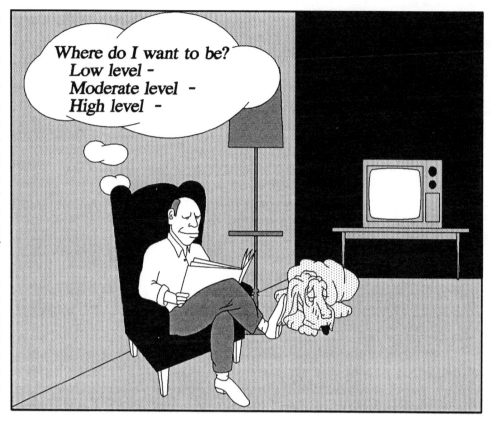

As I have stated earlier in this book, I believe that the two- or three-minute walks you've been taking can be beneficial to your health. But to be completely honest, I am not certain that **optimal** health and fitness benefits can be gained with these short bouts of exercise. In order to insure health and fitness improvements, I think it is wise to add a few longer sessions to your exercise plan.

My final exercise recommendation is to try to incorporate at least two ten-minute walks on most days. I think that if you can do this five or six days a week and maintain your schedule of a few two-, three-, and five-minute daily walks, you will achieve the moderate level of physical fitness discussed in earlier chapters.

Recall that in our studies at the Institute for Aerobics Research, the all-cause death rate in moderately fit men was 26 per 10,000 while the rate for low fit men was 64 per 10,000. The corresponding figures for women were 16 in the moderately fit and 40 in the low fit. Thus, it seems worthwhile to get at least into the moderately fit category. For those of you who are already moderately fit, there is some further benefit in doing a bit more and achieving the high fit category. In our study, the high fit men and women had all-cause death rates of 20 per 10,000 and 7 per 10,000 respectively. You can decide if the reduced risk of early death in the high fit group, or having a higher level of functioning, is worth the extra effort.

Establishing the Ten-Minute Walk

How can you increase some of your shorter walks to 10 minutes, or add one or two 10-minute walks to your daily schedule? Only you can know what approach is most likely to result in success. You may find it easiest to stretch some of the shorter walks, perhaps at lunch time or in the morning. It may be easier to simply maintain your present schedule of walks and find a new time when you can add a 10-minute walk. Or, if you are not now taking a walk with a family member or friend after supper, this might be a good time to add a 10-minute walk. This would give you a good opportunity to discuss the events of the day, try to resolve any family problems or issues, or simply visit.

Below, please list up to three times a day when you will take a 10-minute walk. If you want to start with one walk per day, that is fine. At this point, no more than three times a day is necessary.

When Will I Take a Ten-Minute Walk Next Week?

1. _____

2. _____

3. _____

4. _____

5. _____

Try to establish the 10-minute walk habit, and maintain the shorter walks that have become part of your life. Over the next few weeks, you should strive to get up to two or three 10-minute walks on most days. You will find some days when it is impossible to carry out your plan, but just resolve to pick it up the next day.

I seldom miss a day of running and virtually never miss two days in a row. But, as I write this on a Saturday afternoon, I missed running on both Thursday and Friday this week. I was able to get back on schedule this morning with a five-mile run with my wife. We plan to run in a 15-kilometer race tomorrow. Exercising has become as ingrained a habit with me as brushing my teeth. I know that if I miss a day or two, I will pick up the schedule at the next opportunity. This is what you should strive for. I'm confident that you can also establish a consistent exercise habit.

MAINTAINING YOUR NEW HABITS

Changing a habit is not as difficult a task as most people think. Mark Twain said, "It is not difficult to stop smoking, I've done it hundreds of times." Obviously, the hard part is maintaining the change once it is made. If you can maintain a new behavior for an extended time, it becomes easier to continue. As stated earlier with the tooth brushing example, once a new behavior becomes routine, you will feel strange if you don't do it.

Two keys to maintaining health behavior change are planning for problems and how you will solve them and making the behavior automatic. I discussed earlier how you can anticipate problems that may interfere with your exercise plans. You may know that you will be quite busy next week, or that you will have house guests. Now is the time to plan how you

Keys to Maintaining Behavior Change

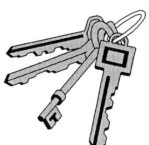

1. Plan for problems and how to solve them.

2. Make the behavior automatic.

will keep up your exercise when next week gets here. Plan to take your guests on a walking tour of your city or take a walk after dinner each evening in your neighborhood. Plan some active recreation with them. You know best how to solve the problem and stay on schedule, but it will probably take some planning.

I have stressed over and over again, the importance of making your exercise routine and a part of your daily life. One way to do this is to reconstruct your perception of yourself in terms of your status as an exerciser. You may have been sedentary for years, and you thought of yourself as sedentary. Now you should think of yourself as an active person who exercises regularly.

There are numerous techniques behavioral psychologists have developed to increase success in maintaining health behavior change. My colleagues, Drs. Kelly Brownell and Judy Rodin, have written a book on weight maintenance entitled *The Weight Maintenance Survival Guide.* I suggest that you obtain a copy of this maintenance manual and adopt some of the ideas in your exercise maintenance program. Brownell and Rodin are two of the nation's leading health psychologists, and they offer many helpful suggestions that you can use.

WHAT ABOUT OTHER ACTIVITIES

Most exercise examples given in this book are for walking. This does not mean that walking is the only activity that is appropriate for your new approach to exercise. I have used walking as an example because it is something that you can do almost any time and anywhere. It requires no skill, partner, or special clothing or equipment. In fact, it doesn't make any difference what you do for exercise as long as you expend the energy. Remember that the energy expenditure calculations described in Chapter 2 give credit for any activity. There are dozens, if not hundreds, of recreational, sports, household, or other leisure time activities that you can use to get you daily exercise dose. I do not believe it is useful for me to give you several detailed lists of activities or a specific exercise prescription to follow. I have used walking as an example, and if you want to do the equivalent in another activity, that is fine.

A convenient way to quantify exercise was developed over twenty years ago by Dr. Kenneth Cooper, who founded our center in Dallas. He published a best selling book, ***Aerobics,*** in 1968, in which he described the Aerobics Points system. This approach simply assigns a point value to a given amount of physical activity. For example, walking two miles at 3 mph yields three aerobics points, and 30 minutes of singles tennis yields two points. I mention this scoring system because the Aerobics Points tables are widely available and can be used to determine the amount of various types of exercise. They also allow you to combine several types of exercise into a common scoring system. This is an alternative approach to the energy expenditure calculations described earlier.

In a previous chapter, I presented results of our research on physical fitness and all-cause mortality. Three fitness categories were described--low, moderate, and high. The number of aerobics points per week that should produce these fitness levels are shown below for men and women.

Average Weekly Aerobics Points		
To achieve:	__Men__	__Women__
Moderate fitness	**18-36 points**	**15-24 points**
High fitness	**>36 points**	**> 24 points**

People 50 years of age and older can probably achieve the fitness levels with points near the lower limit of the range for a given category. Younger persons need to do a bit more. Thus, if you are a 30-year-old woman and you want to develop a moderate level of fitness, you should strive to get 20 or more points a week. If you are a 60-year-old man, 38 points will probably get you into the high fit group.

Some of you may chose to increase your activity level by taking part in a sport, and that's fine too. I have nothing against sports as a form of exercise. Participation in most sports requires a bit more planning and time than if you walk for exercise. You should do what works for you. Of course, you can also integrate sports, walking, stair climbing, and other activities routinely into your day.

One advantage of sports is that they may require you to use other muscle groups and may help maintain muscular strength and flexibility (depending on the sports you select) in addition to the aerobic benefit. Although I have stressed aerobic exercise and its health and functional benefits in this book, I do think it is important to develop and maintain musculoskeletal fitness as well. It's a good idea to do some strength and flexibility training in addition to your aerobic activities. This can be done with formal weight training sessions, calisthenics, or by doing vigorous muscular work around the house and yard.

ADDITIONAL REINFORCEMENT

I made some recommendations in a previous chapter on how to reinforce your new exercise habits and how to seek social support. You should think about additional techniques for reinforcement and additional sources of support. One thing you may wish to consider is the Fit for Life award system. The Institute for Aerobics Research developed this approach as part of the national fitness program we developed for school children. Several different awards are used in the program.

The Fit for Life award was designed to be implemented in the home instead of at school, and it can be used by the entire family. The award is to recognize commendable exercise behavior. You are given an exercise log to record your (and your family's) exercise participation. Self-recording and completion of the log is the responsibilty of each individual. The logs can be returned to the Institute and an award selected.

There is a modest charge for the awards, and a wide variety of awards are available. If you think this system might help you or your family members maintain exercise behavior, please contact the Institute at the following address and request information about the Fit for Life award program.

Institute for Aerobics Research
Youth Fitness Division
12330 Preston Road
Dallas, Texas 75230

SOME CONCLUDING THOUGHTS

A reporter asked me the other day, "Why should I exercise?" After thinking a moment, I replied, "It will make you feel better, function better, look better, and live longer." And, upon reflection, I still think that is a good answer. Exercise is indispensable to good health and a high level of functional capability. There are a few things you can do to add as much quality to your life. Our data show that a 65-year-old man who is physically active has the functional capacity of a 40-year-old man who is sedentary. That is a tremendous advantage. There is no pill or other medical intervention that can provide so much advantage in terms of ability to meet daily responsibilities. Moreover, it is unlikely there will ever be another intervention that has comparable effects to regular exercise.

I would like to see the entire U. S. population exercising the equivalent of at least 30 minutes of brisk walking each day. I believe the result would be a terrific improvement in the public's overall health and our national productivity. But you shouldn't wait for the rest of the nation to adopt regular exercise habits. Make your move now, and begin to enjoy the benefits. Good luck.

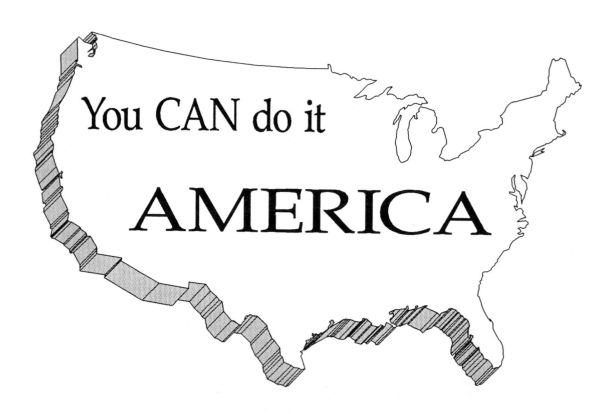

Appendix A

MET VALUES FOR SELECTED PHYSICAL ACTIVITIES

One MET is the energy expended by your body while you are resting quietly. Energy expenditure of any activity can be expressed as a multiple of resting expenditure. Thus, an activity of three METs means that you are spending energy (calories) at three times your resting level.

The method of monitoring your daily caloric expenditure presented in Chapter 2 requires you to record the number of hours of activity you got for the day in each of three intensity categories: moderate (3 to 4.9 METs); hard (5 to 6.9 METs); and very hard (7 or more METs). This appendix shows the intensity category for several common physical activities based on their MET requirement.

Some judgment is necessary in using this table because the MET cost of an activity can vary depending on circumstances. For example, walking at 3 mph requires an energy expenditure of 3 METs when walking on a firm surface on the level. If you walk at 3 mph in soft sand at the beach or up a steep hill, the MET value may be as high as 6 or 7 METs.

Doubles tennis requires 6 METs on the average, and is listed as a hard activity in this appendix. But it is possible to play doubles tennis so slowly that it requires less than 5 METs, and should be scored as a moderate activity. Conversely, you could play so vigorously that 7 or 8 METs of expenditure would be needed.

Remember that your honest and subjective rating of exercise intensity can be accurate, especially after you get some experience. If an activity seems about as intense as walking at 3 to 4 mph (15 to 20 minutes per mile), it should be scored as a moderate activity. If an activity is as vigorous as jogging, it is a very hard activity. If an activity seems to be harder than walking but not as vigorous as running, score it as a hard activity.

Moderate Intensity Activities (3-4.9 METs)

Calisthenic exercise	Snorkeling
Carpentry in workshop	Softball
Golf (not riding a cart)	Table tennis (recreational)
Horseback riding	Vacuuming carpet
House painting or paper hanging	Volleyball (recreational)
Mowing lawn (not on a riding mower)	Walking at 3-4 mph (15 to 20 minutes per mile)
Raking lawn	Weeding and cultivating in the garden
Sailing	Weight lifting

Hard Intensity Activities (5-6.9 METs)

Aerobic dance

Basketball (non-competitive)

Carpentry outside

Construction work
 --doing physical labor

Digging in the garden

Doubles tennis

Downhill skiing

Fishing (wading in stream)

Hiking

Hunting (small game, walking)

Scuba diving

Skating, ice or roller

Snow shoveling (dry snow)

Square, folk or fast dancing

Stair climbing (moderate pace)

Swimming (slow pace)

Walking at 4.5-5.5 mph

Water skiing

Very Hard Intensity Activities (7+ METs)

Backpacking (hilly country or rough trails with a heavy pack)

Basketball, soccer, singles tennis, or racquetball (competitive)

Cross-country skiing

Mountain climbing

Rope jumping

Running

Stair climbing (fast pace)

Swimming (fast pace)

Very hard physical labor

Appendix B

TESTING YOUR KNOWLEDGE
ABOUT EXERCISE QUIZ

The following are the explanations and answers to the "Testing Your Knowledge About Exercise Quiz" on page 25.

1. *False*   Humans vary on all traits, including metabolic rate. The causes of these variations are not well understood. But, even if you do have a relatively slow metabolic rate, exercise will cause an increase in caloric expenditure and will contribute to weight loss.

2. *False*   It may be easier to eat 100 calories than to burn 100 calories through exercise, but the accumulative effect of exercise can increase caloric expenditure by several hundred calories per day. Remember that exercise provides many positive benefits aside from energy expenditure.

3. *True*   Exercise maximizes the loss of fat and can help prevent the loss of muscle. In fact, exercise can build muscle tissue.

4. *True*   How far you go is more important than how fast you go. It is not the rate of caloric expenditure that is important in weight loss, but the total number of calories that are burned. If you prefer to burn calories at a slower rate by walking instead of running, the effect on weight loss will be the same. Of course, running will get the job done faster!

5. *False*   The rubberized "sweat suits" and other fancy gimmicks do not provide any benefit. In fact, they may cause you to overheat, especially in warmer weather. Wear clothing that is comfortable for you.

6. *True*   Climbing stairs is an excellent way to burn a lot of calories. It is so strenuous that you will not be able to climb continuously at a fast rate unless you are very fit. You can accumulate significant caloric expenditure over the course of a day if you regularly take the stairs rather than the elevator.

7. *False*   Your resting pulse rate will decline as you become more physically fit. This is a sign that your heart is getting stronger and can pump more blood with each heart beat.

8. *True*   Improvement in fitness is related to the frequency, intensity, and duration of exercise. In the past, many people have overstated specific combinations of these variables that must be achieved to obtain certain health benefits. You should not worry about achieving a specific dose of exercise, but focus on increasing your activity level. Even modest increases in activity will, over time, produce changes in fitness and provide other benefits as well.

9.   *True*   Unfortunately, "spot reduction" just does not work. Your body adds and removes fat according to genetic and hormonal factors. You must concentrate on increasing caloric expenditure and achieving a negative caloric balance. When you do this, you can reduce fat in general, but you cannot control the areas where the fat will be lost.

10.   *True*   Jogging and cycling are excellent aerobic exercises and are ideal for many dieters. They provide both psychological and physical benefits. They burn a lot of calories quickly, make improvements in overall physical fitness, and make you feel good. Lower intensity activities such as walking also make important contributions to fitness, health, and weight control; but it may take a little longer.

11.   *True*   Most people have access to stairs, so it is easy to add several flights to your daily routine. Look for opportunities to build stair climbing into your day.

12.   *False*   Due to technological achievements, there is much less occupational physical activity today than there was 200 years ago. Motorized transportation and countless labor-saving devices have greatly reduced activity on the job and in leisure time.

13.   *False*   If anything, exercise will temporarily blunt your appetite, although in the long-run, more exercise will require more calories. However, exercise seems to help regulate caloric intake to appropriate levels. Regular exercisers weigh less than their sedentary peers.

14.   *False*   Caloric restriction causes significant loss of muscle tissue. Weight lost by exercise or by a combination of exercise and diet, tends to come predominately from fat stores.

15.   *True*   Building small incremental activities into your daily routine can have significant benefits in both weight loss and weight maintenance programs. The total accumulation of energy expenditure is what is important to weight loss efforts. Strive to accumulate several activities over each day.

The LEARN® Education Center

The LEARN Education Center was established to respond to the increasing demand for scientifically sound, state-of-the-art publications, training courses and services. The Center is dedicated to the continuing development of health and wellness materials, including audio tapes, newsletters, professional training guides, leadership training programs, and professional counseling services.

Publications currently available from The LEARN Education Center are as follows:

The LEARN Program for Weight Control by Kelly D. Brownell, Ph.D.

The LEARN Program Monitoring Forms

The LEARN Programs Cassettes by Kelly D. Brownell, Ph.D.

Making a Weight Loss Program Work - The LEARN Program Leaders Guide by Kelly D. Brownell, Ph.D.

The Weight Maintenance Survival Guide by Kelly D. Brownell, Ph.D. and Judith Rodin, Ph.D.

The Personal Maintenance Kit by Kelly D. Brownell, Ph.D. and Judith Rodin, Ph.D.

The Weight Control Digest - Professional Edition

The Weight Control Digest - Consumer Edition

Living With Exercise by Steven N. Blair, P.E.D.

Ordering Information

This manual and the other materials distributed through The LEARN Education Center are not available in bookstores. You may write or call the number listed below to obtain current pricing and shipping charges. Discounts are available for bulk orders.

For your ordering convenience, a toll free number is availabe and may be called 24 hourse a day. Payments can be made with your MasterCard, VISA or by mailing your personal check. You may also fax a copy of your purchase order. All orders are shipped with 24 hours of receipt, and next day and second day delivery service is available.

As you use our publications, we sincerely welcome any comments you may have that would make these materials even better and we encourage you to tell us how we are doing.

For ordering or general information, please write or call us at:

The LEARN Education Center
1555 W. Mockingbird Lane, Suite 203
Dallas, Texas 75235

Our toll free number is (800) 736-7323
In Dallas (214) 637-7700
Our fax number is (214) 637-0529